DE MY STI FY

THE SCIENTIFICITY OF HOMOEOPATHY

RAJAN DUBEY

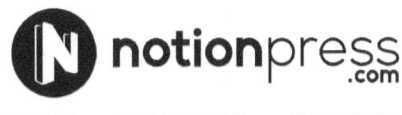

INDIA · SINGAPORE · MALAYSIA

Notion Press

Old No. 38, New No. 6
McNichols Road, Chetpet
Chennai - 600 031

First Published by Notion Press 2019
Copyright © Rajan Dubey 2019
All Rights Reserved.

ISBN 978-1-68466-921-9

CONTENTS

ABOUT THE AUTHOR

Dr. Rajan Dubey, a coherent thinker, a research-based author and a renowned physician, has always expounded and encouraged the substantial correlation that Homoeopathy and science retain.

Since the very beginning, he has always abided by the teachings of Dr. Samuel Hahnemann. He holds a distinct healthcare vision and has been renowned for over a decade in the field of Homoeopathy for his approach of Holistic Healing.

A scientific researcher, his writings have always been evidence-based and were highly acknowledged since his very first book, *True Perception of Chronic Diseases*. Two of his gross pathological cases were published in an internationally-acclaimed homoeopathic journal *Interhomoeopathy* in June 2014, and they received worldwide admiration.

He is a far-sighted man who always wanted to surpass the aperture by building a bridge and reaching the underprivileged areas facing a paucity of medical services, which led him to establish his trust – 'Medigene Homoeopathic Research and Development' (MHRD) in 2012. MHRD primarily focuses on empowering the necessitous cancer patients in a holistic way, i.e., a state of physical, mental and social well-being. His work has been eminently appreciated, and he has also been felicitated at Belgaum National Conference in 2011. Also, he was honoured with the Award of Achievement by Dr. Arun Bhasme (Senate member, Maharashtra

University of Health Sciences) at the Mega HomoeoCon, in 2018, for his outstanding work and contribution in the field of Homoeopathy.

In clinical practice, he holds great expertise in resolving gross pathological cases with his chiselled knowledge of Medicine as well as *Materia Medica*. Bestowing this knowledge to homoeopaths all across has been his invariable undertaking, by virtue of this firmly-held belief:

"A candle loses nothing by lighting other candles."

INTRODUCTION

"Experience is the only teacher we have. We may talk and reason all our lives, but we shall not understand a word of truth until we experience it ourselves."

– Swami Vivekananda

Being a medical student teaches you a lot more than the mere functioning of the human body. It all begins the day you enter the corridors of your medical college wearing a starchy white apron, the stethoscope on your shoulders and with different aspirations in your eyes. I recall my earlier days of coming across exciting and challenging subjects like Anatomy, Physiology, Biochemistry and dissection of cadavers in the formalin-scented laboratories. The latter was the experience of a lifetime that no medical student can ever forget. Amidst all this came the most spine-chilling subject – 'Organon of Medicine,' which left me in a very baffled state. Its comprehension was a constant tussle all through my years of homoeopathic college life. This was more so because of the absolute failure of correlating theory with practicality in the former years of student life.

Many thoughts and questions over-crowded my mind as to why our Founder, Dr. Samuel Hahnemann, even came up with these concepts of miasm and chronic diseases, but these soon assumed a backseat in my mind. All these dormant thoughts came back to life in the final year of my college when I chose to work on miasms as my topic for the thesis.

That was when the process of researching began, and it only became more pronounced once I stepped into the practical world.

A medical student, whose mind is too fragile for all the baggage to be lifted, breaks his shell of medical college and enters into the medical world to explore it, where he is rocketed with new and varied theories. Having faced similar bombardment, the very first thing that I could vividly remember was the first aphorism stated by our Dr. Samuel Hahnemann in his *Organon of Medicine*: **"The physician's high and only mission is to restore the sick to health to cure as it is termed."**

Once into the outside world, this mission now seemed like an illusion.

This transition that my life encountered led me to commence a process – a process of learning, experiencing, experimental study and also a process of endowing students with the experiences I encountered on my way, thus paving the way towards healthy healing with Homoeopathy and also outspreading Homoeopathy.

All through this process, I could disinter that our body always tries to retain a state of homeostasis which is kept in place by the many feedback mechanisms working continuously in our body. Having known this, I always wondered as to how such a harmonious and meticulous functioning of our body could ever be disturbed? How does the body fall victim to incessant chronic diseases? What causes disruption in our bodily homeostasis at the level of the cells and proteins? Is it just environmental influences or emotional setbacks, or is it something more?

Like the saying goes, I finally realised that there's more to it than meets the eye, only after reading through Dr. Hahnemann's *The Chronic Diseases*, which held a key to all of my uncertainties. Having unravelled the concealed knowledge after great many efforts, I always pondered over how wonderful the easy comprehension of this knowledge in the former years of my college life would have been. Unfortunately not being so, I resolved to outspread this knowledge to a majority of the people, be it the tenderfoots or even the most experienced people.

These aspirations led me to write my very first book, *True Perception of Chronic Diseases,* to break all the myths about miasms and also to portray the scientificity of Homoeopathy. Moreover, the book also rendered an insight into the evolution of Earth, the origin of miasms as well as chronic diseases, their classification and also the practical utility of miasms with case presentations.

Not silencing my deepest intentions of imparting knowledge, my second book chiefly focuses on how the process of chronicity sets in and incapacitates the human body. How does our life-governing vital force function and how does it fall victim to the insults of factors from both within and without?

Also, this book intends to scientifically prove and clarify '*The Theory of Chronic Diseases,*' which was proposed by Dr. Samuel Hahnemann back in his era. The modus operandi followed for this was a retrospective study of 30 subjects selected from a pool of around 10,000 patients who visited Medigene Homoeocare, our clinical institute located in Mumbai, and were suffering from chronic diseases. This was accomplished by tracing the journey of disease from their childhood to present day in a chronological order during the process of case-taking. Among these, 10 cases are explained in complete detail to serve as a practical guide to the readers. Also, an insight into the remedies holding close proximity to the case and the differentiation between them has been imparted.

All through my journey, which still has a lot to unfold, a crucial lesson that I shall embrace for a lifetime is: **"Learning is a constant process of discovery – a process without end."**

1 | AN INTRODUCTION TO THE BIOPHYSICS OF THE HUMAN CELL

The human body is composed of trillions of cells. Each and every cell in itself is a representation of the whole body and corresponds wholly to it. Each cell incorporates a variety of organelles that are assigned with specified tasks.

Certain examples of the same can be the nucleus of the cell containing within itself the genetic material, the mitochondria being termed as the powerhouse of cells, or the cell membrane constituting a protective layer to the cell. These organelles are functionally equivalent to the diverse organs that our body encompasses. Every function that our body performs is also expressed by each and every individual cell. Thus, we can rightly infer that the human body and each of the cells are analogues of each other.

Just like humans, each individual cell possesses the faculty of analysing each and every stimulus that the micro-environment, which they reside in, impresses upon them. On analysis of these stimuli, the cells select an appropriate behavioural response so as to ensure their survival. Furthermore, the cells also have the ability to assimilate and learn from the environmental experiences that they come across, and create cellular memories, which they even pass on to their progeny.

A practical illustration of this is the infection of the body with a virus. The immune cells come into play to produce protective protein antibodies against this virus. To accomplish this, the cells create new genes to serve as a blueprint in the fabrication of the protein antibodies for the virus. The genetic memory of this antibody is preserved within the cells so that the body instantaneously launches a protective immune response on being exposed to the same virus in the time to come. The new cells formed by cell division receive these genes and the associated memory from their ancestor cells. A pattern akin follows in the working of the entire body.

Whenever our body is exposed to a stimulus from the environment, it tends to scrutinise it and reacts with a behavioural response apt for its survival. It also retains a memory of it to deal with similar future confrontations.

To elucidate this better, consider a child who touches a hot pan for the first time. Being unaware of the consequences, the burning sensation and pain on touching the pan lodge in his mind as a distinct memory and, henceforth, even looking at the pan would release certain neurotransmitters from his brain that cause a sensation of unease. As a response, the person now becomes cautious while handling a pan, until he finally comes to realise that it is only when the pan is hot that it can cause discomfort and pain. This new memory soon makes place in his brain, and his reactions change accordingly. To that effect, I could now fully perceive that the cells as well as the whole body create memories based on their lifetime experiences and react in a way that is best suited for their endurance. I could thus finally come to terms with why Dr. Hahnemann has time and again directed us to treat everyone in a holistic way, i.e., considering the person as a whole.

I further came to acknowledge the fact that every cell is made up of four types of organic molecules, namely, polysaccharides, proteins, lipids and nucleic acids (DNA & RNA). Although all of them are exceedingly important, proteins surpass them by virtue of being the building blocks of life.

The year 1953 was a milestone in the field of science due to the discovery of the double helix, the twisted-ladder structure of the deoxyribonucleic acid (DNA) by Watson and Crick. Since then, it has been a firmly-held belief that only genes have command over all the functions and structures of our body. My mind always pondered that if this was to be true and if only genes had control over the working of our body, wouldn't we all fall prey to similar diseases that we inherit from our ancestors? Wouldn't only a single disease then run through the entire family from generation to generation?

Puzzled by all of this, I came across a famous quote, which read, *"Nail the basics first and detail the details later."* This led me to return to the basics where I reread into the process of protein synthesis which occurs in two steps, viz. transcription and translation. These steps are, in turn, kept in check by regulatory proteins (gene regulatory proteins) that control the synthesis of proteins in a cell. Scientists have also come to recognise that external factors such as the environment where we reside, our thoughts and emotions, the nutrition that our body receives, drugs & chemicals, etc. are efficacious in influencing our regulatory proteins, thereby playing a potent role in altering the biochemistry of our body. Thus, we can rightly deduce that it is not only the genes alone but also the external factors that play a role in the functioning of the human body.

Initial predictions claimed that the human body encompasses more than 1,00,000 genes – one gene for every individual protein synthesised in our body. However, as a result of the constant research, we can now understand through the Human Genome Project that the body contains an estimate of only around 25,000 genes. Newer studies reveal that these 25,000 genes can however express themselves in at least 30,000 diverse ways via the regulatory proteins. And as we have already inferred that these regulatory proteins are also influenced by external factors, we can rightly claim that a part of any disease process can be explained by the multitudinous external factors to which our cells are exposed.

This is the very scientific foundation as to why homoeopathic case-taking is so comprehensive—beginning from the very childhood and extending till the present age of the individual. Through this, we try to search for the causative factor and the reaction of the individual to them, which can be elicited from the environment the person has lived in since the beginning, the emotions which he has been exposed to and many other external factors, the conjoint effect of which brings about a transformation in the expression of the DNA.

Dr. Hahnemann has clearly stated in Aphorism 5 of *Organon of Medicine* that, "Useful to the physician in assisting him to cure are the particulars of the most probable exciting cause of the acute disease, as also the most significant points in the whole history of the chronic disease, to enable him to discover its fundamental cause, which is generally due to a chronic miasm. In these investigations, the ascertainable physical constitution of the patient (especially when the disease is chronic), his moral and intellectual character, mode of living and habits, his social and domestic relations, his age, sexual function, etc., are to be taken into consideration."

Here, he explains that in the case of acute as well as chronic diseases, exciters play a pivotal role in influencing our gene expression, and he has attributed the environment, emotions, dietary factors, etc. as the exciters. Thus, Dr. Hahnemann could even in that era—250 years ago—fully comprehend the role of external factors as exciters and maintainers of the disease process, which today's scientists attribute to the concept of *epigenesis* (above the genes). In addition to the exciting cause, he has also mentioned the 'fundamental cause,' which according to him is the chronic miasm.

Our body always tries to retain *homeostasis,* i.e., maintaining all bodily functions and structures in perfect similimum. This is ensured by the various, intricate feedback mechanisms that are constantly working in our body.

Our body cannot easily fall prey to chronic diseases by the insults of such external factors. There is something much deeper and detrimental that predisposes our body to chronic diseases. The fundamental cause of chronic diseases is miasm, which further paves the way towards an incessant process of chronicity.

But how exactly does this miasm creep in and weaken our body? How does it lead to such a daunting process of chronicity? What impact do the external factors have on our body? Can we overcome all of these and cure the patient eternally?

2 | THE MISUNDERSTOOD VITAL FORCE

Most of us seem to have an intuitive notion about force. Aristotle, a Greek philosopher, intended to establish the concept of force, but his ideas were not widely accepted.

Two millennia after Aristotle's time, Isaac Newton laid the foundation of laws of motion in response to force. In our day-to-day life, we come across many forces. They can be frictional, muscular, buoyant, electric, magnetic, nuclear, tension in a rope, so on and so forth. Furthermore, a cardinal force responsible for the harmonious functioning of our body, which preserves life, was proposed by Dr. Hahnemann in Homoeopathy, under the title of 'vital force.' You will all be amazed to know that all of the aforementioned forces in nature are governed by four fundamental forces, viz. gravitational force, electromagnetic force, strong nuclear force and weak nuclear force.

These fundamental forces play an important role at the level of atoms and molecules, whereby electrons are kept in an orbit around the nucleus by virtue of the electromagnetic force. On the other hand, protons and neutrons are bound together to form a stable atomic nucleus by the strong nuclear forces. Furthermore, weak nuclear forces are responsible for an interaction between subatomic particles that cause nuclear decay, and they also play an essential role in nuclear fission. The force that holds molecules together is intra-molecular force, which is an electrostatic force of attraction.

Having comprehended the functioning of each of these fundamental forces, we can now infer that the vital force stated by Dr. Hahnemann is a conglomerate of these fundamental forces.

Dr. Hahnemann had unambiguously stated that the vital force is dynamic in nature, present everywhere in the body and is of paramount significance for normal functioning and maintaining the healthy condition in a harmonious way. However, this question has always afflicted my mind: if everything in this universe is made up of atoms, how can we differentiate between the living and non-living?

I came to understand that the chemical processes occurring in living organisms involve the making and breaking of the bonds. This further results in either liberation or absorption of energy, which constitutes the process of metabolism. These processes aid in maintaining life. Hence, the living state and metabolism are synonyms. The living process is a constant effort to prevent attaining equilibrium. It is this metabolism which distinguishes the living from the non-living.

Thus, vital force is not only an amalgamation of the four fundamental forces but also comprises the chemical processes (metabolism) occurring in our body. This differentiates the living from the non-living, which is clearly stated in Aphorism 10 by Dr. Hahnemann: "The material organism without the vital force is capable of no sensation, no function, no self-preservation; it derives all sensation and performs all the functions of life solely by means of the immaterial being (the vital principle) which animates the material organism in health and in disease."

Therefore, we can infer that despite the lack of scientific evolution, Dr. Hahnemann could rightly perceive and introduce the concept of vital force. Sadly, it was misapprehended in those times.

3 | DEMYSTIFY: THE GENESIS OF CHRONIC DISEASES

Around 250 years ago, in the primeval era, Dr. Christian Friedrich Samuel Hahnemann, a German physician, best known for creating the system of medicine called Homoeopathy, accomplished a great task by simplifying the concept of chronic diseases. He also enlightened us on how we can surmount the chronicity in a person and thereby treat chronic diseases.

After 12 years of extensive research, he gave us an insight into the true nature of chronic diseases, whereby he introduced *the concept of miasms* and declared that, "The true chronic diseases are those that arise generally from a chronic miasm, which is the fundamental cause of majority of chronic diseases."

Although medical science had not reached its zenith during Dr. Hahnemann's time, he could still fully comprehend and introduce the classification of chronic diseases. He classified them into **Miasmatic & Non-miasmatic diseases**. **Chronic miasmatic diseases** were further classified into **venereal-originating** & **non-venereal-originating** chronic diseases, based on their source of infection.

Of these, chronicity arising from non-venereal origin—which he termed as 'Psora'—was considered to be the most contagious, destructive and hydra-headed, as its precursor can easily be transmitted by any and every means. Furthermore, diseases arising from Psora tend to change forms and may reappear with a different name and after a few years with a different set of symptoms, thus making it difficult to get rid of the chronicity that had once set in.

Dr. Hahnemann has clearly mentioned in his writings that of all chronic diseases, 7/8th appear to be arising from non-venereal origin, while the remaining 1/8th arise from venereal origin.

Non-miasmatic diseases were further classified as **pseudo-chronic diseases** and **artificial chronic diseases**. The diseases which people incur by continuous exposure to avoidable noxious influences such as indulging in liquors or other dissipations, residing in unhealthy localities, especially marshy districts, etc. are known as pseudo-chronic diseases. These states of ill-health can disappear spontaneously under an improved mode of living, provided no chronic miasm lurks in the body (Aphorism 77– *Organon of Medicine,* 6th edition). On the other hand, artificial chronic diseases are those that are artificially produced by allopathic treatment by the prolonged use of violent, heroic medicines in large and increasing doses by the abuse of calomel, corrosive sublimate, mercurial ointment, etc. (Aphorism 74 – *Organon of Medicine,* 6th edition).

In this contemporary era, we see that a majority of the diseases that are tormenting mankind are chronic diseases when compared to epidemic or sporadic diseases, which were rampant in the past. Nowadays, the treatment appears to be focused more on treating the end-products of chronic disease (Hypertension, Diabetes, etc.) rather than trying to disinter their origin. By virtue of this, we can only eliminate the present conditions rather than the original root cause from which various ailments emanate. On tracing this root cause, the whole process of chronicity can be brought to a standstill. To understand the genesis of chronic disease, we need to comprehend the basic unit of an organism – **the atom.**

As we all know, the basic unit of all structures in this entire universe is nothing but atoms. Each atom is composed of neutrons and protons, which are present in the nucleus, and electrons, which revolve around the nucleus in different energy orbits. Thus, every atom has its own energy. Therefore, we conclude that everything in the universe from the human body to mere dust particles consist of energy.

Energy is defined as the capacity to do work. The two principle forms of energy are potential energy and kinetic energy. Chemical energy is a form of potential energy stored in the chemical bonds of compounds and molecules. Thus, each and every molecule in the body possesses potential energy.

Law of conservation of energy states that, "Energy can neither be created nor be destroyed. It can only be converted from one form to another." Thereby, potential energy is converted into kinetic energy, which allows us to work. This conversion takes place by means of chemical reactions. For every chemical reaction to occur, the requisites are different concentrations of reactants and different temperature conditions.

In order to maintain the life process, the body temperature and concentration of molecules in the body fluids remain subtle for most of the chemical reactions. Any deviation from normalcy raises the temperature and number of reacting particles in the body, which in turn increases the rate of collisions, thereby increasing the rate of chemical reactions. This would then pose a threat to the cells of our body. To reconcile this, catalysts come into play. Enzymes are the most important catalysts in the human body, which are proteinaceous in nature. As our body is mostly made up of proteins, we ought to know about their basic structure.

Proteins are made up of amino acids, of which there are 20 different types. Each protein differs from the other depending upon the sequence of amino acids, which in turn is controlled by genes. This amino acid sequence, known as polypeptide, folds into its characteristic and functional three-dimensional structure from a random coil. This assembled form of protein is termed as 'Native conformation,' which performs biological functions within.

Proteins have four levels of structural organisation in their native conformation:

> Primary structure
> Secondary structure
> Tertiary structure
> Quaternary structure

Since our bodily functions are carried out and controlled by proteins, only exogenous proteins (of miasmatic and non-miasmatic origin) have an ability to disturb the homoeostasis of our body.

These exogenous proteins (antigens) can be in the form of:

> Infectious diseases (venereal & non-venereal; miasmatic)
> Chemicals (non-miasmatic)
> Antibiotics (non-miasmatic)

Whenever any exogenous protein enters our body, an adaptive immune response develops against it, which tries to clear this foreign antigen from our body. But when this infectious agent produces an antigen that is very similar to that present on our normal tissue cells, then it becomes difficult for our immune mechanism to eliminate this foreign antigen, and a sustained response occurs, as the antibodies stimulated to react against the foreign antigen also recognise the similar self-antigens. Hence, the two antigens are said to be cross-reactive. Thus, the auto-antibodies stimulated by the external antigen can cause serious damage to our body.

Following are the illustrations of the same:

> Streptococcal bacteria that causes rheumatic fever produces antigens that are cross-reactive with those on the heart muscle membrane. Thus, the antibodies that react with the bacteria also bind with the heart muscle membrane, thereby causing damage to the heart.

> In Chagas disease, the trypanosomes that cause the disease produces antigens that are cross-reactive with those present on the surface of specialised nerve cells that are responsible for the orderly contraction of the muscles of the bowel. Thus, the antibodies directed against these trypanosomes also interact with the nerve cells, thereby disrupting the normal bowel function.

> One of the immune-mediated causes of haemolytic anaemia appears to arise after an infection with mycoplasma pneumonia where auto-antibodies are directed against certain antigens present on the red blood cells. These are probably induced by a similar antigen present in the microbes.

> Chronic disease arising from abuse of medicaments – sustained administration of certain medicaments for several months produces auto-antibodies that further lead to haemolytic anaemia. Such medications contain anti-hypertensive, alpha-methyldopa, quinine, sulphonamides, penicillin, etc.

Our body has been endowed with a strong defence mechanism to withstand all insults to maintain its equilibrium. So, it does not easily fall prey to chronic diseases. However, there are certain criteria where the body has a predilection to develop chronic diseases, which are as follows:

1. Frequent episodes of acute infection.
2. Hindrance to the normal healing process in the form of chemicals or antibiotics.
3. Antigen being homologous to the normal cell.
4. Infective organism resists the host defence and persists in the organism for a longer duration, leading to chronic disease.
5. Inflammatory agents, which are foreign to our body, such as silica dust, metal, wood splinters, etc., cannot be removed.

When any infection, chemical or antibiotic, enters our body, an adaptive immune response occurs – due to which there is change in the pH and temperature of the protein environment, which occurs due to the inflammatory response. As we all know, proteins are flexible-linked peptide bonds between the amino acids, which enable the protein to adopt a variety of shapes by the rotation and flexion of amino acids.

The factors that determine the shape of protein are:

1. The sequence of the amino acids.
2. The interaction of the electromagnetic charge amongst the linked amino acids.

Most amino acids have a positive or negative charge, which acts like a magnet. Like charges cause the molecules to repel one another, while opposite charges cause the molecules to attract each other. Change in the pH and temperature due to the above mentioned factors causes change in the electromagnetic force between the amino acids in turn leading to change in the structure of the protein.

If such changes occur frequently and persist for a long duration, a gradual disruption tends to occur in the protein structure, and it loses its three-dimensional shape called native conformation, which results in protein-misfolding. This further leads to the protein going into an inactive state. This disruption can only be reversible as long as the primary structure of the protein is retained because the amino acids are still intact and not yet separated. So, it can refold to its normal structure and return to its normal environment. However, it can also go into permanent denaturation, which is an inactive state of the protein, which is the precursor of multiple chronic diseases in our body. For example, Alzheimer's disease, Parkinsonism, Cystic Fibrosis, Neurodegenerative Disorders, etc. Such repeated insults leave a residual effect in the organism, disturbing our bodily equilibrium and thus leading to chronicity.

To substantiate the scientificity of the *Theory of Chronic Diseases* proposed by Dr. Samuel Hahnemann even in today's era and also to facilitate its easy and practical utility, we took up a retrospective study. The methodology involved a retrospective study of a random sample of 30 patients from a pool of around 10,000 patients who were suffering from different chronic diseases and who had visited Medigene Homoeocare, our clinical institute located in Mumbai.

The purpose of the study was to trace down the precursor that led to the chronicity in each patient.

Among these, 10 cases are explained in complete detail to serve as a practical guide to the readers. Also, an insight into the remedies holding close proximity to the case and the differentiation between them has been imparted.

NEURODEGENERATIVE DISEASE: A TACITURN MAIDEN

DR. RAJAN DUBEY

Towards the end of the year 2012, we received a call for a home visit, as the patient, a 20-year-old girl, was unable to walk on account of her paralysis diagnosed as neurodegenerative disease.

We always tend to explain to our patients the process of the first consultation with regard to case-taking and the required time span. The outcome of this was realised when we reached her residence and met a girl with an inanimate face. She seemed absorbed in herself and soon handed us a written note denoting her troubles. On asking to justify her action, her mother explained that she had always been uncomfortable expressing about herself and thus she preferred to pen it down.

We could deduce the following from the matter received from her and from our personal interaction, where she said, "Since the age of 12 years, I have always had the complaint of recurrent aphthous ulcers. In the last 2 years, this has increased. Because of this, it is difficult for me to eat or even drink anything. Also, since the past 2 years, my menses have been irregular." Furthermore, with water welled up in her eyes, she said that the watering from the eyes had been a constant complaint since long as well.

On asking her to elaborate about each ailment in detail, we discovered that she had been operated thrice for fibro-adenoma of the breast. It all started with sudden amenorrhea at the age of 18 years, and she was also diagnosed with bilateral fibro-adenoma of breast at the same time. On enquiring more, we were astonished to know that every time she went under the knife, her menstrual irregularities would settle, only to be again followed by the fibro-adenoma, which was later diagnosed as benign phyllodes tumour.

The major concern for the patient was her not being able to walk or even get up from bed. Elucidating it, she mentioned how it began with her leg pain, where she used to lose her balance and felt like falling on her left side. She had difficulty in standing as well. The pain was more in her left leg.

She used to end up using her right leg more to compensate for the pain and then that also began hurting. Her legs used to ache a lot, especially her heels. Both her legs were swollen, and she could not sit with her legs folded. Also, as she could not lie on her back, she had to lie on either side. Whenever she used to do that and stretch her legs, it was painful. The leg pain made it difficult for her to get up from the bed. She had to sit for at least 5-10 minutes before getting up, that too only with some support. All this gradually started after being operated for fibro-adenoma for the third time, which took place in December 2011.

Explaining the previous complaints, she said that she was having difficulty in eating as well, due to mouth ulcers. Ever since childhood, she had been very fussy about food—be it vegetables, non-vegetarian food or fruits. She only had food that she liked. There were times when she only had tea along with bread and biscuits. She did not like to have food from someone else's plate. Also, she could not tolerate anyone touching her belongings.

She further continued saying, as a kid, she was not very fond of playing and that she only liked watching television. Now she does not feel like doing anything. Her body had become very weak, and she did not even feel like getting up. Her sleepiness had increased in the past two years as well.

Her mother added to this by saying that she used to always complain of leg pain and that her gait was also affected. This was noticed only after she was operated for the fibro-adenoma. Moreover, since September 2012, her left leg used to get twisted following which she could not walk at all. She also said that her daughter was unable to control her urge for urination, so much so that when she slept on her abdomen she passed urine involuntarily.

On a detailed interrogation of the evolution of her troubles, we could trace that at the time of birth she had aspirated meconium, which had led to Pneumonia. She had been an overweight baby, with birth weight of more than 3 kilograms. She then contracted chickenpox at the age of 12 years in 2004. From her birth till the age of 12 years, she did not suffer from any major illness, other than constipation.

It was in 2006 that she noticed the greying of her hair.

In 2009, their family had shifted and was now staying in a joint family. Later on in 2010, she had irregular menses and was then diagnosed with fibro-adenoma of bilateral breast, which was operated on in September 2010. After this, the patient got her regular menses in October 2010, but was again diagnosed with fibro-adenoma, and this was again resected. This process continued for 3 consequent times until 2012. Further, we could actually pinpoint that in January 2012, after being operated for the last time, the weakness, pain in the legs and disturbances in her gait were noticed. In August 2012, she had to bear the news of the sad demise of one of her cousins. And by September 2012, she again started complaining of amenorrhea and even inability to walk.

On asking her to describe her persona, she mentioned that since the very beginning she did not like anyone touching her, be it her father when she was little or her friends in college. She did not like people touching her possessions either, which was why she would even ask her mother to wash her hands before touching any of her belongings. She would warn them that whatever they wanted, they should ask her for it and she would hand it over. They did not need to touch her things.

She did not like it when her mom washed her hair. She tended to get angry if hot water was used for bathing, as she further stated that it made the leg pain worse. She had always had a liking for dancing and watching TV serials and became angry if her mom said no to her watching them.

The mother contributed to the conversation by saying, "My daughter doesn't like it much here after we shifted. She has also started getting angry, especially when she is alone. When I am around, she feels better." While we were still discussing this, the patient distracted us by saying, "I have always been afraid of my mother. She used to hit me when I was a child. She also used to lock me up in the room. She never allows me to act according to my will." Continuing further, the mother added that before shifting, while in their old residence, her daughter used to roam around and would be with everyone. But in the new house, because of the fights, she would say they should not stay there.

Now she did not like going out at all. Even if all the family members were going out, she would say they could lock her in the house and leave. She said, "I can't even walk now." If anyone asked her about this, tears would well up in her eyes and she would be unable to speak. Only when someone initiated conversation would she talk. She did not even talk to her cousins. She wanted all her things to be in the proper place. Her mother narrated an instance where the patient had asked one of her younger cousins to pick up something from the bed and keep it in its proper place. To this, he abruptly replied that his father had bought the bed. Ever since, she had stopped asking him to do any work.

Throughout the narration, it was observed that the patient was very reluctant – even while explaining her chief complaints. After much digging, she appeared to somewhat open up, and she admitted that ever since childhood she had been a reserved person. She did not like talking much. She initially liked to roam around, but after shifting homes that too had stopped. When she mentioned that she was not too keen on making friends, her mother hopped into the conversation. She added how her daughter did not share her feelings with anybody except her and that too sparingly. She continued to mention how she avoided meeting new people and when amidst them she hardly spoke. She then added that her stubborn daughter did not like her brother much and never allowed him to touch or use any of her belongings. If he scolded her, she scolded him back.

To this, the patient snappishly said that she got angry whenever her brother did such things. Further, the patient added that she did not like to stay in her new house because there her aunt did not treat her properly. The discrimination between her and her own children disturbed her. When asked more about it, she seemed to avoid the topic with tears in her eyes. On asking the reason for her tears, she side-lined it by stating that it was simply due to the dust in the air.

■ MENSTRUAL HISTORY:

Amenorrhea since 2010, which was better intermittently after fibroid removal. But since 2012, again amenorrhea

Cycle: Irregular/4 days, red, no clots. Offensive

No complaints before, during or after menses

Leucorrhoea: Occasional

■ PHYSICAL GENERALS:

Appetite: Good, could tolerate hunger

Likes: Spicy food

Dislikes: Sweets

Thirst: Thirstless

Perspiration: Scanty

Urine: No complaints

Stools: Constipation

Sleep: 8-9 hours. Refreshing. Occasional salivation during sleep

Dreams: Could not remember

Fears: Fear of falling

Thermals: Could not tolerate summer; comfortable in cold weather. Hot patient

■ EXAMINATION:

Sensory	Right Lower Limb		Left Lower Limb	
	Upper Leg	Lower Leg	Upper Leg	Lower Leg
Pain (Pin-Prick)	Present	Present	Present	Present
Light Touch	Present	Negative	Present	Negative
Temperature	Present	Negative	Present	Negative
Position Sense (Proprioception)	Present	Negative	Present	Negative
Vibration Sense	Present	Negative	Present	Negative

Motor	Right Lower Limb	Left Lower Limb
Knee Flexion (Hamstrings)	Grade 3	Grade 3
Knee Extension (Quadriceps)	Grade 3	Grade 3
Reflexes	Right Lower Limb	Left Lower Limb
Knee Reflex	Brisk (3+)	Brisk (3+)
Ankle Jerk	No Response	No Response
Babinski	Extensor Response +Ve	Extensor Response +Ve

■ SUMMARY OF THE CASE

It is a well-acclaimed declaration by the medical fraternity that neurodegenerative diseases are incurable – which was our conjecture as well, until a young girl approached us who was initially unable to walk and later landed up in a paralytic state. A hallmark of neurodegenerative diseases is the formation of misfolded protein aggregates that cause cellular toxicity and contribute to cellular proteostatic collapse, whereby leading to degeneration and death of the nerve cells. Proposed causes for degenerative nerve diseases include genetic and environmental factors such as being triggered by a viral infection like Herpes Simplex, Epstein Barr, Varicella Zoster, etc., which can induce alterations and degeneration of neurons both directly and indirectly. Similarly in our case, the precursor was chickenpox, i.e., Varicella Zoster, which the patient suffered from at the age of 12 years, whereby posing a future threat for overgrowths as well as nerve degeneration. Thus, we can classify this as a miasmatic disease of non-venereal origin, i.e., Psora (For details of the Journey of Disease, refer to Chart no. 16).

One of the hindrances while case-taking is an encounter with reticent patients, such as ours. She was non-expressive, sad and had an inanimate face. Even as a child, she was reserved and reluctant to make friends and meet new people. She was disinterested in going out with her family, yet a fear of being alone prevailed where she always wanted her mother around. As a person, she was averse to any of her family members touching her or her belongings, so much so that she even asked her mother to wash her hands before touching any of her possessions. Experiencing inequity between herself and her brother by her aunt made her upset. Moreover, she got vexed when she was refrained from watching her favourite television serial. Over time, she appeared to enter into a state of indifference, which was a gradual process and could be perceived only after understanding the case in all of its aspects.

Very few rubrics led us to a remedy, which worked wonders in this case.

▮▮ Rubrics considered were:

> ➤ Mind; TALK, indisposed to
> ➤ Mind; INDIFFERENCE apathy, everything to
> ➤ Mind; COMPULSIVE disorders
> ➤ Mind; TIMIDITY
> ➤ Mind; CONTRADICTION intolerant of

The remedy prescribed was Conium Maculatum. Conium proved to be the most suitable remedy, as the course of the disease was slow and gradual, which constitutes an important aspect of the remedy, as it cannot be thought of in manifestations which are sudden and violent.

One of the eminent features seen in the remedy is of 'weakness due to over exertion,' which shows itself on both the physical as well as the mental plane.

Talking about the mental faculty, the Conium state arises after an emotional setback like incessant grief or anxiety (which is a form of mental exertion). This eventually leads to mental weakness resulting in slow and gradual breakdown of the intellectual faculty whereby comprehending and thinking skills become sluggish. In this state, the mind gives out, and even the slightest mental exertion affects the patient adversely, and gradually he progresses towards a state of imbecility. On the physical plane, there is progressive weakness due to over straining, which gradually leads to paralysis.

Thus, the slow and gradual progress of the disease eventually results in imbecility and paralysis on the mental and physical plane respectively.

The longstanding mental trauma is ensued by a depressive state where they develop an aversion to people, society, relations, etc., yet an interesting irony is that they fear solitude.

Another feature of the remedy is being very particular about trifles, which ranges to the degree of obsession. On the emotional plane, they are very sad and discontented with everything – which slowly and gradually advances to a state of indifference, thereby making case history difficult to extract from the patient.

In my years of clinical practice, I have seen this remedy hold a great utility in non-miasmatic cases where a physical injury has led to a gradual process of degeneration. The other remedy which came close was Sepia Officinalis. However, in Sepia, the indifference is directed towards loved ones arising from a long standing history of being abused, domineered or contradicted, whereas in our case, the indifference was reflected in a generalised way. Thus, Sepia was ruled out.

Although 'Fear of being alone, yet desires company' persists in both Conium and Sepia, the only difference was the exciter as also understanding the component of indifference in its full length.

An important lesson that this case fetched me was that remedies appear to be closely-knit in some of their facets, which makes them look alike. However, the key to disinter the similimum lies in perceiving each and every aspect of the patient as also the remedy in complete detail.

▋▋ REMEDY PRESCRIBED:

Conium Maculatum 200, 1 powder daily for 3 consecutive days from 26/11/2012.

▋▋ FOLLOW-UPS:

22/12/2012

- ➢ Able to stand but only in a bending posture and with support.
- ➢ Not able to straighten her legs.
- ➢ Able to walk with support since the last 15 days.
- ➢ Swelling over the right leg still present.
- ➢ Also complaining of back pain recently.
- ➢ Pain in the lower abdomen: Both iliac fossa since the beginning of December. Pain extended to both the legs.
- ➢ Sensation of urine and stools restored, but control had not been established yet.
- ➢ Appetite had improved; now ate well.
- ➢ Weight had increased.
- ➢ Menstrual history:
  Last menstrual period: 15/12/2012
  Flow for 2 days.
  No significant complaints during menses.

▋▋ PRESCRIPTION: Placebo

30/01/2013

- ➢ Last menstrual period: 11/01/2013
- ➢ Tingling sensation in both lower limbs

➤ Unable to sit

➤ While sleeping, folded her legs towards her abdomen

➤ Could not move her feet

➤ Urine frequency had increased

➤ Constipation

▋ PRESCRIPTION: Placebo

01/03/2013

➤ Last menstrual period: 07/02/2013

➤ Pain in lower abdomen extending to the legs still persisted with the same intensity.

▋ PRESCRIPTION: Conium Maculatum200 one dose

17/04/2013

➤ Last menstrual period: 20/03/2013

➤ Leg pain and swelling – cried with pain

➤ Urine frequency had reduced

➤ Constipation still the same. Ineffectual urge. Did not pass stools for 4 days. Had to strain. Had to do manual evacuation of stools

➤ On examination: Bilateral pitting pedal oedema

▋ PRESCRIPTION: Conium 200 one dose

10/12/2013

➤ The patient seemed to improve gradually but did not get menses in the month of July 2013

➤ August 2013 – menses on 11th August

➤ No menses in the months of September, October and November

➤ Last menstrual period: 01/12/2013

▊▊ PRESCRIPTION: Placebo

The patient was gradually improving and was on placebo throughout 2014. There was improvement in her gait, and she could now walk and stand, although not independently but with minimal support. The control over bladder and rectum was completely established. She was started with physiotherapy and dietary advice as an auxiliary mode of treatment. Her menstrual cycles showed slight irregularities intermittently, which did not require any interference.

In 2015, improvement continued until August when she complained of recurrence of the lump in her right breast.
18/08/2015

> Last menstrual period: 23/07/2015
> Menses were regular now
> Pain in the left heel
> Blackish discoloration over the left foot. No itching. Occasional watery discharge
> She complained of pain in her leg, extending from the right iliac fossa, but now only during physiotherapy
> Heaviness in the abdomen. Passed flatus
> Constipation. Passed stools in 4-5 days. Also, pain in the anal region. Because of this complaint, she refused to walk
> Recurrence of lump in the right breast in the upper, inner quadrant. On examination, it was a non-painful, mobile lump

▊▊ PRESCRIPTION: Placebo

She was advised not to take treatment in any form for the lump.
21/11/2015

> Last menstrual period: 17/11/2015
> The eruption over the left foot had increased since 2-3 days. Watery discharge

> Pain in left iliac fossa, only in squatting position and during exercise
> Mouth ulcers occasionally, especially before menses
> Constipation was better; passed stools every alternate day
> Since the start of winter, there was pain in the legs and also burning sensation in the right leg
> While walking, could not touch the heels to the ground
> The lump in the breast was still the same. There was no pain

▋▋ PRESCRIPTION: Placebo

Gradually, she could now climb up the stairs, but descending the stairs was still not possible. Intermittently, she experienced imbalance in her gait. Her menses were regular now, with a rare skip in the cycle.

In 2016, she visited us in the month of October.

14/10/2016

> She was much better now
> The size of the lump in the right breast was still the same
> Last menstrual period: 09/10/2016
> Swelling over the feet had disappeared
> There was a corn on the left heel, which was painful on pressure
> This time there was much improvement in her gait, and she could walk without support. On asking, she said she could also jump and also did so. She could bend forward and now sit on the floor and also get up

▋▋ PRESCRIPTION: Placebo

The patient was better since then. She could walk better now without any support, with a slight imbalance.

The menses were regular. The lump in the right breast was still the same.

The most recent follow-up was as follows:

18/05/2018

- ➤ Last menstrual period: 22/04/2018
- ➤ Now walking on her own. One incident where she had a fall, no injury. But after this she was again complaining of burning in the right leg
- ➤ No aphthous ulcers
- ➤ Lump in the right breast – no change

The patient is still on continuous treatment with us.

CASE 2

HYPERTHYROIDISM: CONCENTRATION DIFFICULT

DR. RAJAN DUBEY

....

One fine morning as I entered my clinic, I came across a middle-aged man with bulging eyes waiting in my visiting area. This gave me a clue to his diagnosis, which was confirmed once he started talking about his ailments.

He complained of having Hyperthyroidism since 2011. He also mentioned suffering from headache and acidity along with burps, which had intensified since the last two years. Acidity and headache often happened when he was not eating on time. He had previously even consulted an Ayurvedic doctor who had suggested him certain food restrictions.

When asked about how his condition was diagnosed, he mentioned how someone had noticed his popped-up eyes and suggested to him to undergo a Thyroid test. He also had a past history of Koch's for which he underwent a treatment for six months. Not being symptomatically better, the treatment was prolonged for one more month. Suddenly after 2-3 weeks of completion of the Koch's treatment, he noticed the bulging of eyes.

On retrieving his history, he narrated that he had taken a loan to buy a luxurious house in 2007-2008. Before buying this house, he used to go to the gym regularly but then eventually he stopped going as the sense of responsibility peeped in. He had come to the realisation that he had to repay the loan soon. He thus became more responsible than before. The amount of the loan was huge, and this was the first time he had taken any kind of loan. The calculations of the loan were always on the back of his mind.

He described himself as a calm and cool person who preferred to analyse each and every situation before reacting to it.

When asked about his childhood, he affirmed that he was the youngest in his family and was always inclined to business-oriented fields. He further added that he was ambitious and had always wanted to do something out of the box. He was pursuing his Bachelor of Commerce but had to leave his studies mid-way due to family issues. He had also joined Chartered Accountancy (CA) in 1990 but could not give his exams. In 1993, he shifted to Mumbai, as he was doing a job there. He rented a house there, and then finally, after undergoing lots of struggle, he finally managed to complete his CA in 1995. He further added that the reason for shifting from Jodhpur to Mumbai was primarily because of less salary coupled with his weak financial background. In Mumbai, he often used to sleep without having dinner, as his mother was not there to serve him food. The initial days of struggle made him strong and practical.

On querying about his ambitious nature, he added that his father was a shopkeeper. He had always dreamt of becoming a businessman. Due to the lack of financial support, he could not start his own business while pursuing CA. He also entered into a partnership with his friend, and they began their own financial company, but it did not work out well.

In the 10th grade, he managed to pass with grace marks. During his 11th grade, he studied and did a job simultaneously, still managing to pass with first division: 63%. His moral got boosted afterwards, and he then developed an image of a sincere and intelligent student in his society. Because of this moral confidence, he had started developing interest in studies. People around him always used to say that he would go on to become successful someday.

As a young child, he was attached to everyone and was well-pampered and protected by his family. He mentioned he was obstinate as a child. He explained his obstinacy by giving an example. Once, his sister and brother-in-law had gone for a movie and they did not take him along with them so he decided not to eat for 3 whole days and further insisted them to watch the same movie again with him. His mom also fulfilled all his demands. He further expressed his nature to be quite different from that of his other siblings. He described himself to be intelligent and ambitious unlike his other brothers who were struggling because they were more into work requiring physical labour.

He described his self-esteem and ego to be very high. He expected a lot of respect. He mentioned that his ego got hurt if someone did not talk to him properly. He considered himself to be superior. For him, he was important and above all.

He expected his colleagues in office to call him 'sir.' If he was not called that, he would feel bad and scold them. A similar incident had already taken place twice at his workplace. He also mentioned that if, for instance, he hired some taxi driver and if that driver did not speak in a desired manner, his ego would get hurt and he would yell at that driver. Right from his childhood, everyone had spoken nicely to him; he simply could not understand the fact how someone could not speak with due respect to the person they were dealing with. He also felt annoyed when his clients did not receive his calls. He further said that whenever he felt bad, he went into his hibernation mode.

He added that he considered himself to be superior in his family and deserved all the due respect because he started and built everything from scratch. Through his constant will and struggle, he had now attained that name, fame and property, which had made him a stronger person and had developed this attitude in him. The initial days of struggle made him so stone-hearted that he did not feel any attachment, any emotion whatsoever. He did not feel like helping anyone, and even if he helped, he did not like to show his emotions. He believed that giving gifts or other presents during any occasion—be it Valentine's Day or birthdays—was simply a waste of time.

He further mentioned that he had a strong feeling of insecurity in his subconscious mind, although there was no major reason to worry. He had never had a protective father. Protection in the sense that if anything happened in the future, there would be no one to support him. He could not afford any mistake and had to be on his toes always, as there was also a loan, which added to the tension. Now his priority and worry point was his 13-year-old daughter's height, as she looked younger than her age (8-9 years). She also had thyroid complaints.

He continued to mention that his nature had become very serious. His subordinates were often scared of his serious nature, as he often scolded them. He further added that the reason for his prompt decision-making nature was just because of the fact that he became independent at such an early age.

Lately, he had been experiencing lethargy and a lazy feeling which was more in the morning and evening. He got tired soon so he preferred sitting to standing. Internally, he experienced a lack of energy. There was also constant leg pain and weakness. Physical exertion drained out his energy. He always felt mentally exhausted and disinterested. He also added that lately he was not able to concentrate even during his business meets. He often lost track of conversation and entered into a different train of thought. He currently felt no passion for the current work and had started losing interest in his business as well as his personal life. In 1996, he joined *satsang* (congregation), which made him feel spiritually connected.

His inspiration being Dhirubhai Ambani, he preferred talking more like a business consultant, and he expressed that if someone were to make him the Chief Executive Officer of the company, he would be very happy and accept it with gratitude.

For him, self-respect was the most important asset. He said it made him feel independent and also that the society treated the person in a better manner. Whenever he used to go for business meets with clients, they often had a perception of him being a salesperson; their body language used to hurt his ego. But he always thought of working hard and decently. He expressed himself to be a positive person who often trusted other people blindly. He further said that there was no insecurity about money. He possessed full capability to do business, which he had dreamt of, and had also started it, but it did not work well.

For him, loud noise caused fatigue, and he preferred a peaceful environment.

A brief history was later taken from his wife where she mentioned that he did not get angry or react. That he believed quite a lot in spirituality. He did not take much tension and was very sensitive but could not express. He was a simple person who liked spending most of his time at home and did not have a dominating nature.

■ PHYSICAL GENERALS:

- ▷ Appetite: Could not tolerate hunger; avoided fasting
- ▷ Thirst: Thirsty; drank water often
- ▷ Perspiration: Moderate
- ▷ Sleep: Good, for 8-9 hours
- ▷ Dreams: Got weird dreams, once in 2-3 weeks but could not remember
- ▷ Stool: Constipation; had to go frequently
- ▷ Thermals: Chilly patient. But also could not tolerate extreme temperatures

■ SUMMARY OF THE CASE

Aforementioned is a case of Hyperthyroidism, wherein a butterfly-shaped gland present in the neck (thyroid) becomes overactive, leading to excessive production of the thyroid hormone. Here, the process of autoimmunity led to Hyperthyroidism, wherein the body produced antibodies (a protein produced by the body to protect against bacteria or virus) called thyroid-stimulating immunoglobulin, which mimic the action of thyroid-stimulating hormone (TSH), thereby leading to excessive production of thyroid hormones.

In this case, the patient had contracted Tuberculosis in the year 2008 before which he was in apparent good health. He then took anti-Koch's treatment for 6 months. Not being symptomatically better, the treatment was prolonged for one more month. For the first time, he observed the bulging of his eyes, which was 2 weeks after stopping the medication during the convalescence period. Thus, we can infer that it was Mycobacterium Tuberculosis which was the precursor that initiated chronicity in the form of Hyperthyroidism. As we are already aware of the fact that Tuberculosis can only be transmitted by the air-borne route, which is a non-venereal route, we can distinctly classify this case as a case of chronic miasmatic disease of non-venereal origin, i.e., Psora (For details of the Journey of Disease, refer to Chart no. 11). As we know, once the chronicity has set in, the body can easily fall prey to various ailments if triggered by an exciting cause.

On analysing the history, the patient as a child was very carefree and stubborn. Although being the youngest of all siblings, he was always fascinated by the idea of becoming a business tycoon. He always had a protected environment. Over the years, circumstances changed and he had to take up responsibilities whereby his then-luxurious life took a turnaround and became a life full of struggle. All this transformed him into a diligent and serious person.

Having struggled through the years, he finally bought a huge house of his own, for which he had taken a loan in the year 2007-08. This created a state of worry for him, which was constantly playing on his subconscious mind. It was this sustained state of worry which acted as an exciting cause.

One of the prominent aspects of the case was his difficult concentration, wherein while being in a conversation he seemed to lose interest and went in his own chain of thoughts. On the physical plane, he complained of feeling lazy, and even the slightest physical exertion drained his energy.

▮▮ Rubrics considered were:

> ➤ Mind; BUSINESS aptitude for
> ➤ Mind; CONCENTRATION difficult
> ➤ Mind; SENSITIVE, noise, to
> ➤ Generals; WEAKNESS, enervation, exhaustion, prostration, infirmity exertion, from agg

After repertorisation, we came to a group of remedies namely Calcarea Carbonica, Kali Carbonicum, Lycopodium Clavatum, Mercurius Solubilis, Natrum Carbonicum and Sulphur. The patient being thermally chilly, Calcarea Carbonica, Kali Carbonicum and Natrum Carbonicum were now in the race.

After having comprehended every attribute of the case, two remedies which closely resembled the case were Kali Carbonicum and Calcarea Carbonica, because of their common aspect of insecurity.

From my clinical experience, I have come to understand that 'tremendous fear of being alone' constitutes the central theme of Kali Carbonicum. They are in a state of constant struggle to attain the security that they always seek. This struggle is seen in the form of the obvious irritability and easy startling.

Also, on considering the patient's disposition, we could deduce that he was a very mild person. Thus, we could rule out Kali Carbonicum.

Calcarea patients are known for their insecurity, which is present even after being nurtured in a well-protected environment. Majority of the times, this insecurity represents itself in the form of various fears like fear of impending disease, of misfortune, of animals, especially of insects. This aspect of fear is also very marked in children. Calcarea children are very obstinate, indolent and have an aversion to play. Generally, Calcarea patients are very sensitive to cruelty so much so that the child cannot even bear the sight of it.

Other facets of Calcarea include a state of being sad and gloomy or even self-doubting. Another tinge seen in the remedy is of suspicion that he is being watched. Intellectually, Calcarea patients are poor in learning and make mistakes while talking.

On the physical plane, Calcarea has an affinity for glandular affections. Also, in this case, the chronicity manifested itself by disturbing the function of the thyroid gland.

Thus, Calcarea Carbonica was prescribed, and favourable results ensued.

REMEDY PRESCRIBED:

➤ Calcarea Carbonica 200, 1 powder on 20/02/2017

FOLLOW-UPS:

10/03/2017

➤ Patient was better than before. His concentration had improved.

➤ Acidity still persisted on and off, with weak digestion. Also, had few episodes of headache.

➤ In the recent days, he complained of a lethargic feeling in the morning.

➤ Investigation done on 09/03/2017 which indicated the following:
  • Serum TSH - 0.006 mIU/L

PRESCRIPTION: Placebo

08/04/2017

➤ His concentration kept on improving gradually.

➤ Headaches were better this time. His acidity and gastric issues had resolved comparatively. Also, the feeling of lethargy was better than before.

➤ This time the investigations read as follows:
  • Serum TSH - 0.017 mIU/L, which was done on 07/04/2017.

▌ PRESCRIPTION: Placebo

17/06/2017

➤ Investigations done on 01/06/2017
  • Serum TSH - 0.019 mIU/L; FREE T_3 - 5.7 ng/dL; FREE T_4 - 22.5 ng/dL
➤ Symptomatically, he was much better than before.
➤ Headache had reduced; frequency was only 3-4 times since the last medicine. He had stopped taking painkillers, which he did initially.
➤ Tiredness and lethargy still persisted with a lesser intensity now.

▌ PRESCRIPTION: Placebo

12/08/2017

➤ The complaints of headache and weakness showed great improvement. Acidity was still present on and off.
➤ Recent Investigations were as follows:
➤ Serum TSH - 0.029 mIU/L; FREE T_3 - 5.9 ng/dL; FREE T_4 - 2.20 ng/dL

▌ PRESCRIPTION: Placebo

15/12/2017

➤ He kept improving gradually, and all the complaints had now settled to a major extent.
➤ Investigations in this month were as follows:
  • S.TSH - 0.032 mIU/L; FREE T_3 - 6.6 ng/dL; FREE T_4 - 22.6 ng/dL

▐█ PRESCRIPTION: Placebo

The patient was keeping well with the remedy, with no repetition required. Also, his anxiety had reduced – which was well indicated with his reducing frequency of getting investigated, which was seen in the beginning.

The recent follow-up was on 28/02/2018

> ➤ The frequency of headache had been very less, only 2 episodes since the last follow-up.
> ➤ The gastric complaints had improved with marked reduction in the flatulence and acidity. Lethargy was much better.
> ➤ He visited the clinic only if he had some ailment. As such, no medicine interference was required, as improvement had initiated and continued.

CASE 3

POLYCYSTIC OVARIAN SYNDROME: A DAMSEL WITH THE TAG "DECEIVE ME NOT"

DR. RAJAN DUBEY

....

In the summer of 2015, a very cheerful and animated girl aged 22 years came to visit our clinic. Once she started expressing herself, her excited self was soon side-lined by the worry of her ailments. This worry seemed to arise from having consulted many different schools of medicine and yet neither of them making any difference in her sufferings.

Her major concern was that she was amenorrheic since the past 5 months. On further enquiry, we came to know that she was a known case of Polycystic Ovarian Syndrome (PCOS) and had irregular menses ever since puberty. Her menstrual history was as follows:

First Menstrual Period (FMP): 7th grade, 12 years of age, menses lasted for 6-7 days.

After that, there were no menses for 9 months. Along with this, she also complained of hair growth all over her body especially over chest, thighs, abdomen and back (Hirsutism). She had taken 3 sittings of laser treatment for the same but later stopped. Furthermore, she also complained of hair loss which started since puberty. Since a year she was also suffering from chalazion on both eyes. It started with the right eye and then to the left. She said surgery was never an option for this complaint, as she had always been scared of needles.

She further narrated that she had always been a fat kid since childhood. She could not wear nice clothes, which was pretty annoying and depressing to her. The thought that she was not normal made her cry, but she preferred not to show it. Even if she had a conflict with her parents, she would never let anyone know. She got very uneasy whenever the thought of her not being normal crossed her mind. It was very upsetting. Initially, she used to constantly ponder over why she was not getting her periods. But since the past two years, she had been going to the gym and also started walking. Her menses were still irregular.

Last year, she had met with an accident and was admitted in the ICU for 5–6 days. But she did not want to stay there because hospitals always reminded her of morgues and spooky silence, which she got to understand from watching movies.

Explaining more she said, initially she used to get angry very easily if anybody said anything to her. She was very aggressive before, always used to be angry. She never needed a specific reason to shout. But in school, she was very introverted. When she was in 12th grade, she opened up a little, and now during Bachelors of Mass Media (B.M.M.) course, she became an extrovert. Now she could talk to anyone. She was cranky previously and stayed mostly at home with her mom. But with the people outside, she used to think before reacting. She would get angry even if anyone touched her.

When she was in school, she had a fear of crowds. She also used to fear boys because she always thought that whatever she said there would always be a reaction. If anyone scolded or shouted at her, she immediately felt insulted. Hence, she did not like to say anything wrong. If she wanted to say that somebody was wrong, then she would frame it in such a way that the other person did not feel negative about it. She would not like something wrong happening to others.

She did not like anyone betraying or lying to her. She narrated the following instance, "When I was in the first year of my B.M.M. course, I had 7-8 friends out of which I was close to two of them, one girl and a guy.

I had a crush on that guy; everyone in college knew that I had a crush on him. But that guy asked my other friend out. I felt very bad at that time. At that time, I did not show my feelings to them, but once they left, and I was alone, it was an outburst, and I cried because they lied to me. I felt betrayed, and I cried for a week. All my friends lasted only for a period of 6 months."

Narrating one more instance where she felt the same, she said, "There were 2 friends who used to be with me only for some reasons. There was a friend who was about to get married in two months but used to be with some other guy telling her parents that she was with me. Also, she lied to me that she was at home while she was not and was roaming with some guy. That time I felt that she lied to me."

She also said that with friends, she gave her 100%. No one could tell something bad about her. Whenever anyone lied to her, she felt betrayed. Betrayed meaning she felt very hurt on the inside. Now, she felt that rather than making such friends, she should just stay alone.

She continued to add that she was in a relationship with someone. He stayed in Bangalore. She had gone for a pilgrimage once, and during that time he had come to Bombay. He met one of her friends, and they had gone for a movie – which she came to know later. She felt bad about that and began interacting less with him. She felt lied to. She was very attached to him. For her, people were important, their feelings were important and not money, car or materialistic things. She was more attached to her family and her fiancé.

During her childhood she was an introvert who never participated in anything because of her fear of crowds. She had to follow rules and regulations at home like greeting everyone and talking politely. If someone shouted or was angry with her, she used to start crying before they even touched her.

She then mentioned how she used to hit her elder brother, as there was always a comparison. He was allowed to go out at night, he always got freedom, and she did not. She was always affected due to this discrimination of gender. She used to feel very bad about it and cry at times. She was complaining by nature at that time. Even now, a single stare from either of her parents was enough to make her quiet. She could never back-answer her father.

As a child, she was very attached to her grandfather. He used to talk very nicely with her and also would stop her mom from hitting her. When she was a kid, she used to bite everyone, so everybody would be scared to play with her. She also used to like instigating people. She added that she liked roaming around in her father's shirt.

Once we were done with the case and she was about to leave the cabin, we were very surprised at her excitement when she shouted "Yeah…" like a child and went out.

On interacting with her mother, she described her as a loving child but also at the same time an angry one. She further said, "She gets into an argument with me and her brother if we speak to her in a higher tone. She gets angry on being teased. In her childhood she was very scared of me. She is a very sympathetic girl; for example, if she passes by a beggar she'll give some money."

▆▆ PHYSICAL GENERALS:

> Appetite: Normal
> Craving: Sweets, ice cream, chocolates and chicken
> Aversion: Nothing specific
> Thirst: Thirstless
> Thermals: Hot patient
> Stool: No complaints
> Urine: No complaints
> Sleep: 8 hours, refreshing
> Dreams: None
> Fears: Extreme fear of needles and reptiles. Also, she was afraid of being in the dark. Whenever she was alone, she felt like someone was behind her

■ SUMMARY OF THE CASE

A noteworthy piece of advice that this case rendered was – "It's the simple things in life that are the most extraordinary and only the wise can observe them."

In our case, we could get glimpses of the patient's childish and vibrant behaviour by her babbling talk. We could not miss out on her strikingly evident gesture of running out of the cabin like a child and screaming "Yeah…" after the case was done.

This gesture provided us a better insight into the case thus teaching us the significance of the skill of observation. Apart from this, a sensitivity which was perceptible throughout was of 'being betrayed,' which she had experienced in different walks of her life, the consequence of which was that her friends did not last for too long.

As a child, she behaved in a quirky manner, be it dressing up in her father's shirt or biting everyone around. Another aspect of her childhood was her feeling of jealousy, out of which she used to bite her brother. Additionally, she also had numerous fears, which could not be over-looked, so much so that when alone she felt that someone was standing behind her.

■ Rubrics considered were:

> ➢ Mind; JEALOUSY general
> ➢ Mind; CHILDISH behaviour
> ➢ Mind; AILMENTS from disappointment, deception

After evaluating the case thoroughly, we came up with a remedy whose sphere of action is primarily mind, brain and nerves, i.e., Hyoscyamus Niger. This remedy is full of intermingled illusions and hallucinations, portraying a maze of symptoms and thus leaving the physician in a perplexed state. This state is outwardly reflected where the patient talks with non-existent people and visualises things.

They always crave the undivided attention of their near and dear ones, the deprivation of which leaves them disappointed and jealous. Such experiences of unhappy love lead them to a dismay of being betrayed, thus paving the way towards mental aberrations.

Their gestures are distinct and can create laughter wherein they nip everyone, smile and talk at length in a foolish way. Although very naïve and foolish, they are intellectual unlike Baryta group who are intellectually compromised.

Defining my conversance of Hyoscyamus patients, they are very vibrant and animated in their demeanour. They are also known for their mischievous behaviour where they tend to instigate people around. They also display a sexual inclination where they talk about sexual matters and also sing amorous songs. Also in the maniac state, they can expose their genitals and fumble with them.

Hyoscyamus patients are burdened by many diverse notions like fear of being poisoned, of being pursued, of being bitten by a cat or dog, of wife being unfaithful, etc. Overall, they are very fearful; they especially fear solitude and also many fictitious fears. All these fears are only the tip of the iceberg of a deep-seated suspicion.

One more segment of the remedy is the vehemence of their anger, which is usually a consequence of their jealousy. The extent of anger is such that they have an impulsive desire to kill.

Lastly, we need to differentiate Lachesis, as both the remedies share a common aspect of jealousy and vindictive behaviour. However, Lachesis is very quick-witted and highly intelligent, and Hyoscyamus can be easily differentiated, as they appear to be foolish and childish in their conduct.

This case was of non-venereal origin, i.e., Psora, as the disease originated from malaria, which transformed over the years leading to recurrent jaundice and ultimately to hormonal disturbances (For details of the Journey of Disease refer to Chart no. 6).

▌▌ REMEDY PRESCRIBED:

> ➤ Hyoscyamus Niger 200, 1 powder on 25/05/2015.

▌▌ FOLLOW-UPS

12/06/2015
> ➤ Last menstrual period: 26/05/2015. Got menses after 5 months.
> ➤ Chalazion on the left eye had now decreased in size, but the one on the right eye was the same.
> ➤ Leucorrhoea since one week.

▌▌ PRESCRIPTION: Placebo

07/08/2015
> ➤ Last menstrual period: 12/07/2015
> ➤ The chalazion on the left eye had completely gone, and on the right had decreased in size
> ➤ Mentally and generally the patient was much better

▌▌ PRESCRIPTION: Placebo

18/09/2015
> ➤ Menses were regular
> ➤ Last menstrual period: 12/09/2015
> ➤ Chalazion on left eye had completely gone. Right eye Chalazion had decreased further in size

▌▌ PRESCRIPTION: Placebo

16/12/2015
> ➤ No menses in the month of October and November. No chalazion on the left eye
> ➤ Right eye chalazion gradually decreasing in size

▌▌ PRESCRIPTION: Hyoscyamus Niger. 1M, 1 powder

22/01/2016
> ➤ Last menstrual period: 21/12/2015
> ➤ Chalazion much better on both eyes

▌▌ PRESCRIPTION: Placebo

02/04/2016
Last menstrual period: 17/03/2016

The chalazion on the right eye had also reduced. She had developed a few rashes on the right hand. She mentioned that she had this kind of rashes a few years back. The rashes settled after some time on their own.

In the month of March 2016, the ultrasonography of the abdomen and pelvis was advised, which indicated the following status:

> ➤ Right ovary measured 3.6 x 3.6 x 2.9cms with a volume of 20.4 cc.
> ➤ Left ovary measured 3.8 x 3.4 x 2.3cms with a volume of 15.8 cc.

She gradually kept improving with slight ups and down in the menstrual cycles.

▌▌ PRESCRIPTION: Placebo

The follow-up in the month of February 2018 was as follows:
13/02/2018
> ➤ Last menstrual period: 26/12/2017
> ➤ Had developed acne on the face
> ➤ Had stopped doing exercise and had gained weight in the past 2-3 months

▪▪ PRESCRIPTION: Hyoscyamus N. 1M, 1 powder

Since then till date, the menses have being regular. Also, the chalazion on both eyes had disappeared. The patient was much better and thus no repetition was required.

In the month of April 2018, the ultrasonography of the abdomen and pelvis was repeated which showed a drastic improvement with the following readings:

> ➤ Right ovary measured 3.8 x 1.8 x 1.3cms with a volume
>   of 4.3 cc.
> ➤ Left ovary measured 3.1 x 2.5 x 1.5cms with a volume of 6.1 cc.

NOTE: The chalazion disappeared in the reverse order of its appearance. After the complete resolution of the chalazion, the regularity of menses was established.

ATTENTION DEFICIT HYPERACTIVITY DISORDER: DO NOT TAKE AWAY MY LOVE AND ATTENTION

DR. RAJAN DUBEY

One fine morning, a worried mother consulted us with the annual report card of her 10-year-old daughter. She was taken aback by the fact that her daughter had scored zero in all her subjects. Unable to comprehend what was wrong with her little girl, she could not contain her anxiety and started with the narration directly. The major concern of the mother's worry was the child's behavioural changes in school, where the teacher complained of the child being very mischievous and restless – something which was never the case earlier.

Being the eldest child in the family, she was quite pampered but at the same time, she had always been an obedient child. Her mother was very disturbed by the remarkable changes in her now, which were previously only limited to poor memory and lack of interest in studies. This was once highlighted by her teacher when she was in the 2nd grade. This time, she had scored zero in her exams and was also very weak in Maths and languages. Her mother further narrated that she had started forgetting things, had become less attentive and also could not handle her own things. This was also observed in school, where she used to snatch the belongings of other kids and kept running here and there. If the teacher scolded her, she kept muttering to herself. She also had started forgetting things. If she told her daughter to get something from the kitchen, she forgot why she had gone to the kitchen.

On further enquiry, it was discovered that the child was already diagnosed with borderline intelligence and Attention Deficit Hyperactivity Disorder (ADHD). Ever since childhood, she also had the habit of bedwetting, for which she was on Ayurvedic treatment. This helped her in reducing the frequency, but the complaint still persisted.

On interrogating about her nature, her mother explained, "As a child, she was always pampered but followed whatever was told to her, unlike now, where she has become stubborn and gets angry very often. If she is told not to go out to play, she gets angry and shouts. She has lost interest in studies and likes watching television; she likes watching family and teenage serials."

She did only what she wished to. She got angry if someone talked against her or she was contradicted. When angry she threw things away. Once while she was drinking water, on being told something she got angry and threw away the glass of water. She was also very mischievous. Once she had thrown her grandmother's spectacles in the fish tank. She also threw food in the fish tank.

A year back, her mother shared an instance where she got so angry that she shouted and threw her clothes on the ground while walking. She always complained to her parents that they did not listen to her. She also mentioned that her daughter was the eldest amongst the four siblings, and she used to fight with one of her brothers most of the time.

"As a person, the child is reserved, very possessive about her things and would get angry if someone took them. Whenever I get chocolates for the kids, she gives 4-5 chocolates to the other kids but always keeps a greater share for herself. She always wants everyone to listen to her, and she wants to be a leader. Also, she was always a person who liked to groom herself, wear new clothes, etc. She has also been very fearful as a child. She cannot stay alone and is very attached to her family. She gets scared in the dark and cannot sleep with the lights off," her mother further said.

On asking the mother to ruminate about her daughter's behavioural changes, she explained that it was only after the age of 2-2.5 years that she had noticed her daughter being hyperactive. Until the age of 2, she was so well-behaved that she used to help her dad by getting his footwear whenever he left for some work.

On enquiring more, as to what had happened around that period of time which could be unusual for the kid, the mother mentioned that she had delivered a son during that time. Also, there was birth of another baby in her family.

■■ MOTHER'S HISTORY DURING PREGNANCY:

During the 3rd month of her pregnancy, she came to know that her husband had an extra-marital affair. She used to get angry but could never express it due to a fear that her husband would get angry and leave her. This fear was constant throughout her pregnancy. Also, her mother-in-law was strict and would shout at her on committing any mistake. She used to suppress her anger and vent it out by crying. During the 6th and 7th month of her pregnancy, she suffered from malaria twice and was admitted for the same.

■■ BIRTH HISTORY:

Birth weight: 1.5 kg (low birth weight) Cried immediately after birth. All reflexes were normal.

■■ MILESTONES:

Crawling: 5-6 months Teething: 8-9 months Walking with support: 10th month Talking: When she grew up, she used to talk slowly

■■ VACCINATION HISTORY:

B.C.G. vaccine was given 1 month, 15 days after birth. No complaints after vaccination.

▮▮ OBSERVATION:

The child was not very interactive, was restless and got angry when her mother narrated any bad things about her.

▮▮ PHYSICAL GENERALS:

- ➤ Appetite: Very less
- ➤ Likes: Butter-chicken, non-veg
- ➤ Dislikes: Tea
- ➤ Thirst: Thirstless
- ➤ Thermals: Chilly patient
- ➤ Perspiration: Scanty
- ➤ Stools: No complaints
- ➤ Urine: Urgency of urination. Bedwetting
- ➤ Sleep: Less; did not sleep during the day

▮▮ SUMMARY OF THE CASE

A synopsis of the above case reveals that the presenting complaints of the child were borderline intelligence and Attention Deficit Hyperactivity Disorder (ADHD) (since 3 years of age) and nocturnal enuresis (since childhood). Moreover, an important aspect of the case was that her mother was afflicted with malarial infection twice during the second and third trimester of pregnancy.

While I was deeply engrossed in comprehending the theory of miasms, this case knocked my door and led me to a complete jittery state. I came to appreciate the studies that have already been conducted which suggest that the red cells infected by the malarial parasites sequester in the placenta, disrupting the nutritional exchange between the mother and the foetus, whereby causing maternal anaemia, premature delivery, intrauterine growth retardation, low-birth-weight baby and even foetal loss. Also, I could acknowledge the fact that babies whose mothers contract malaria during pregnancy would later suffer from ailments, including but not limited to learning difficulty and depression.

Thus, in this case, we could deduce that the repeated malarial infection in the mother during pregnancy was the fundamental cause that led to chronicity in the child in the form of neurological-developmental delay, which manifested itself as 'nocturnal enuresis.' Hence, this can be termed as a chronic miasmatic disease of non-venereal origin, i.e., Psora (For details of the Journey of Disease refer to Chart no. 23).

An overview of the case suggested that being the only child in the family, she was the 'apple of the eye' of everyone and was brought up in an extremely pampered environment. In spite of this, she keenly brought her father's footwear whenever he left for work. This gesture showed that she was an obedient child. This was observed until the age of 2.5 years after which there were abrupt behavioural changes in the form of becoming stubborn, getting angered very easily, especially on being contradicted and throwing away things in anger. Academically also she began losing interest in studies and started forgetting things.

A retrospective approach led us to the conclusion that the emotion of 'jealousy' was evoked after the birth of a new-born in the family, wherein all the love and attention was stolen by the new-born. Thus, jealousy acted as an exciting cause and was responsible for aggravating the disease in the form of behavioural changes like hyper activeness and learning difficulty.

While case-taking, it was observed that the child was very shy and was avoiding eye contact. She was also reluctant in initiating any conversation, but her face expressed anger whenever her mother narrated any negative thing about her. This indicated that the child was timid and at the same time was sensitive to criticism.

▮ Rubrics considered were:

➤ Mind; TIMIDITY bashful

➤ Mind; SENSITIVE, reprimands, criticism, reproaches, to

➤ Mind; AILMENTS from anger, vexation

➤ Mind; JEALOUSY General

▌▌ OTHER RUBRIC CONSIDERED:

Mind; JEALOUSY General children in, when a new baby takes the attention of the family away

On repertorisation, the differential remedies that came up were Calcarea Carbonica, Ignatia Amara, Natrum Muraticum, Pulsatilla Nigricans, Nux Vomica and Staphysagria, of which Ignatia Amara and Staphysagria held resemblance with the case.

Taking into consideration every facet of the case, we could understand that the major crux of the case was sudden deprivation of the love and affection due to the birth of a new-born in the family. It was this void that aroused the emotion of jealousy and led to the behavioural changes, whereby an otherwise obedient and mild child displayed paradoxical behaviour by becoming hyperactive, mischievous and angry. This differed from the essence of Staphysagria, which is about dignity and respect.

Although both remedies share a common aspect of being oversensitive, Staphysagria suppresses his anger because of being highly dignified whereas Ignatia cannot express itself, by virtue of being highly emotional. Thus, we could rule out Staphysagria.

Having studied Ignatia through the years, we can perceive that Ignatia are oversensitive and diligent personalities, which is conveyed by their 'delicately conscientious' conduct. This behaviour is not only limited to their work but is also seen in relations where they put an enormous effort. But if someone pinpoints their flaws or hurts them, they become immensely upset and disappointed, as they are highly sensitive to criticism. This heightened sensitivity is also seen on being contradicted, where even an advice is taken as a contradiction.

This in turn leads them into a state of 'silent grief,' where they become reluctant to express themselves. The outward reflection of this could be seen in the form of their changeable mood where one moment she appears sad and the very next cheerful. Another remarkable reaction is their hysterical behaviour, which may be seen through their sudden, unaccountable fainting. (Rubric – Mind; HYSTERIA mild, gentle, yielding, although whimsical and introverted). Being a paradoxical remedy, I have encountered varied reactions where they also sometimes appear to be very mild and calm, which is clearly stated in the rubric – Mind; MILDNESS complaining, bears suffering, even outrage without.

■ REMEDY PRESCRIBED:

➤ Ignatia Amara 200, 1 powder on 17/03/2009

■ FOLLOW-UPS:

Within a span of a few months:
➤ Her mother said she was much better now. Whatever she studied, she could recollect it well. Her intellect was improving.
➤ Bedwetting – 4 times in the last one month.
➤ Her behaviour was also changing; she was getting more irritated. But her teacher was happy with her improvement.

■ PRESCRIPTION: Placebo

17/07/2009
➤ She had her menarche 2 months back
➤ Last menstrual period - 11/07/2009
➤ Bedwetting had reduced. She was also not as mischievous as she was earlier. She obeyed whatever we told her
➤ She had heavy flow during her menses, for which she was advised an Ultrasonography of the pelvis

▌▌ PRESCRIPTION: Placebo

21/08/2009
> ➤ The Ultrasonography was normal.
> ➤ Last menstrual period - 11/08/2009. Flow continued for 7 days.
> ➤ There was improvement in her studies. She scored better in the last exams, though she failed in 2 subjects. But marked improvement in her intellect could be seen.
> ➤ 2 episodes of inter-menstrual bleeding.

▌▌ PRESCRIPTION: Placebo

29/09/2009
> ➤ Menstrual complaints were better.
> ➤ But this time her mother complained that she did not listen to anyone. She had started behaving mischievously again. Recently, her grandmother scolded her when she was not at fault, which made her angry.

▌▌ PRESCRIPTION: Placebo

09/12/2009:
> ➤ This time she had scored 41%, whereas last time she had scored 31%.
> ➤ She still got angry and fought with her siblings when they did not listen to her. She still behaved obstinately.

▌▌ PRESCRIPTION: Placebo

26/02/2010
> ➤ Showed a remarkable improvement where she scored 65.13 % in her exams with improvement in the overall intellect also.

MENORRHAGIA: THE PLEASANT PORCH SLUMBER

DR. RAJAN DUBEY & DR. VAIDEHI MANKAR

A 45-year-old female once visited our clinic. She was accompanied by her daughter, and as soon as she entered, she kept lying down on the sofa till she was called in for taking down her medical history. On asking her why she had been lying down, she said she was feeling extremely weak and was also feeling breathless. The patient then mentioned that she had a fibroid problem for the past 3-4 years, for which she underwent allopathic treatment. However, the problem started again in September 2016.

In February 2016, the patient had got operated for Cerebrospinal Fluid (CSF) rhinorrhoea. The daughter said that she was discharged after 2 months, and within a week, she got meningitis and was again admitted in a homoeopathic hospital for 14-15 days. She was better thereafter. She was also diagnosed with Diabetes Mellitus at the same time.

CSF rhinorrhoea on 11th February 2016 – "I had severe headache as if someone was hitting it hard with a stone, along with vomiting, and I fainted at that time. People said that I was conscious and would run to open the refrigerator door or go outside the house, pass urine in the balcony, but I don't remember anything from those 2 days. When I was taken to the hospital I gained consciousness. I had sneezing since morning and watering from nose."

"After this, I was better for a few months until September 2016 when I was again diagnosed with uterine fibroid. The bleeding was profuse with clots (4-5 pads/day)." She had an urge to pass copious amounts of urine but only a less amount was passed, which was troublesome. There was spasmodic pain while passing urine. She could actually feel the fibroid which was protruding with her hand. Also, she complained of passing stools once in 3-4 days with lot of difficulty which was black, hard with burning pain after passing stools. She felt weakness after the complaint of bleeding had started since 13 March 2017. Before that she had gone to a religious place where she had to climb 100 steps, which she could comfortably do without any breathlessness. "Since the day bleeding had started I experience weakness, vertigo and headache. In the months of January, February, I was absolutely alright. I have acidity complaints since 1999, when my daughter was delivered, which has increased now."

"I feel like a fireball within, with nausea and headache. I avoid talking to people at that time. I feel relieved by medicine (Tab Lanzol-3 tablets/day, since 1999). Also now I have pain in epigastric region. I can't tolerate any tight clothing (undergarment), feel suffocated and have difficulty in breathing so I prefer to wear loose clothes."

"As of now I feel irritated if someone asks me the same question repeatedly. I reply by shouting at the person and tell them not to talk. Even if health-related problems are asked, I get irritated and tell them to let me rest."

"I had been admitted in Sion Hospital; I have become irritable since then. If people ask the same question I get angry. I wonder why they ask the same question repeatedly; if it's my problem, I would solve it. And what do people want to do by asking the same question repeatedly, as the answer won't change. If anyone else asks me about health like my sister or sister-in-law I don't get irritated, but if my husband or daughter asks I get really irritated and want to shut their mouth. When alone I would be listening to songs, and I like it if my friends come to visit at the hospital. In the past 4-5 days I don't feel like eating anything or cooking; whenever I get vertigo

I lie down. By nature, I am jovial and frank. I have a friendly bond with my daughter, and if she likes any guy I don't scold her but behave like a friend."

Childhood: "I had low interest in studies and more in playing. I liked reading story books and gossiping with my friends and spending time with them. I like talking a lot and listening to old songs, soft music of the 60s–80s era. We are 3 siblings; I have two brothers. I was close to my younger brother and did all mischief with him. We were scared of our elder brother. I can spend my entire life along with my younger brother."

"I got married in 1993, I did not want to marry at that time but because of my mother, I got married. After marriage, I was staying at my home with my mother, and my husband would visit me frequently. He works at the Coca-Cola Company. I was never too attached to my husband; instead I am attached to my younger brother and mother. If my mother told me not to visit any place, I would never go against her will. Nobody forces me for anything, and everything in the house is according to me."

"My mother's demise affected me grossly. My life was devastated after her death. I don't have anyone with me after her. Only because I have children, I am surviving. Otherwise my world would have ended. I had no desire to live anymore. Since one year I have become so emotionally attached to my younger brother that if he has any problem I get a headache, vertigo and weakness, and I am in bed thereafter. People to whom I am close I want them around most of the time."

"My mother had heart disease and a high level of blood sugar, and the doctor had said she wouldn't survive for a long period of time. My elder brother made his mind to not put money behind her treatment, as it would be useless. Since then, I did not talk to him, as I was hurt. It seems money is more important to him. Because of him, I lost my mother. Whenever I am in pain, I still remember her. I see her in my dreams too. In dreams, she caresses me and asks me how I am doing."

"My father wanted only male children, so I never got his love or attention. He would take my elder brother along with him. He never spoke to me properly; my mother said he even poisoned me with Tick 20.

Currently, I don't feel any emotion towards him. Anyway, he never loved me. But no father can poison his daughter, so I was hurt and started developing hatred towards him. I neither talk about him nor let his death affect me."

"I don't love my elder brother, and there was hardly any conversation between us. Only to show respect I would talk, but after my mother's death I have developed hate for him. I shall not even attend his funeral. He stays nearby, but I don't even feel like talking or looking at him."

"In my illness, I am afraid of injections, pain and operation. It will be better if I die. I will have to take bed rest; my kids will have to do house chores. I have no fear of operation but of injections; it is quite painful."

History from daughter: "She is very friendly; she mixes easily with everyone and talks. She loves freedom and has given us freedom too. She likes cooking, makes new delicacies and also watches cooking shows. She likes music. Her mood is irritable only when she is into worries. Now she is scared after hospitalisation that she would suffer from a bigger disease or undergo hospital procedures. After her CSF rhinorrhoea complaint, her perspective towards health has changed; she informs us slightest things and has become very careful. Before admission, she was not that health conscious. When healthy she is very jovial and fun loving and plays with kids. She does not like staying at home or staying alone, it makes her irritable. She has many friends; people in the locality of all ages know her very well. She likes dressing up, trying new clothing styles and wearing gold. Likes eating fish, even if it is stored for 4 days, and likes bitter gourd. She does not like *kaju katli* (an Indian sweet), and feels nauseated, even on hearing its name."

"She is close to a few people only. When she is ill, she always wants someone beside her. If she is alone she thinks a lot, and she cries a lot over trivial issues. She does not take any decision without consultation; she is 30% strong and 70% soft by nature. But when we are in trouble she remains strong."

▮▮ PHYSICAL GENERALS:

> ➤ Appetite: Low since 2-3 days
> ➤ Thirst: Thirstless
> ➤ Perspiration: Profuse on forehead, neck and back
> ➤ Sleep: Reduced since 8 days; slept at 2-2:30 am and woke up at 4 am
> ➤ Dreams: Occasionally, only of mother
> ➤ Light: Did not like bright light; kept dim light at home
> ➤ Noise: Irritation
> ➤ Height: Fear when looking down even from the 4th floor; felt as if she would fall
> ➤ Thermals: Hot patient

▮▮ Obstetric history:

$G_2 P_2 A_0 L_2$ female child – 23 years old; male child – 18 years old; both were born full term, normal delivery at hospital.

> ➤ Observation: Did not make eye contact; constant fidgety hands.

▮▮ SUMMARY OF THE CASE

A momentous learning this case has rendered is that we often tend to be misguided by the objective symptoms that patients put forth. The same would have been the situation had we not probed and understood the disease pathology in its finer aspects.

Likewise in our case, the patient was lying down continuously during the consultation, due to debilitating weakness, which was a consequence of anaemia, which had risen from profuse bleeding (menorrhagia). Weakness was so immense that she was compelled to lie down to get relief, as she complained of vertigo even in the sitting posture.

Her family described that in the recent time, due to her illness, she had become so ill-tempered that even their mere questioning made her irritable. Otherwise, she was a very affectionate person who was emotionally dependent initially on her mother, the demise of whom left a void, and now she was dependent on her younger brother.

One of the strange aspects that we came across was her feeling of nausea even if anyone uttered the words 'kaju katli.' Such exaggerated emotions were also seen where even if her near and dear ones fell ill, her health would also get affected.

On conversing with the patient, an interestingly important detail that we found was her fondness for open air, due to which she slept in the balcony.

▮ Rubrics considered were:

> ➤ Vertigo; LYING while amel
> ➤ General; AIR open amel
> ➤ Mind; TIMIDITY bashful

We could understand and sum up the entire pathology of the case in a single pathological general rubric, which was:

> ➤ General; ANAEMIA blood, from loss of metrorrhagia, menorrhagia, menstrual derangements, from

The remedy prescribed was Pulsatilla Nigricans, one whose domain of action is the mind and also works wonders at every juncture where the level of the female hormones becomes disproportionate.

'Changeability' is one of the key features which is evident physically where their pain is of the 'wandering' type as well as mentally where one moment they appear gay and the very next tears well up to whatever you say. Be it their childlike excitement where they love being caressed or on the contrary their sadness where they are easily discouraged.

Mild, gentle and yielding conduct is a recompense for their sensitivity of being mortified. There is a constant internal turmoil where they fear the slightest humiliation. Also they exhibit a few other fears like fear of being alone, of dark, of ghosts, etc.

Their extreme sensitiveness is also reflected where even the slightest deprivation of attention makes them feel lonely. Whenever offended, one of the pre-eminent reactions is weeping easily. When they are not keeping well either physically or emotionally, they are easily irked especially on frequent questioning. Occasionally, they also tend to answer only with the nod of their head.

Another notable fragment of the remedy is that they take religion to the extent of fanaticism where they become over cautious and follow religion very stringently. They adhere to their ideas so rigidly that even the presence of the opposite sex is threatening and the act of sexual intercourse is considered a sin. Their fixed ideas are also reflected in relation to food, where they imagine that certain foods are not good for the human race.

Pulsatilla children cling to their mothers, and cuddling and kissing their loved ones are often seen in their gestures. They have a fondness for being caressed, which is also seen in adults. One of the confirmatory features of the remedy is: Patient feels better when consoled and craves sympathy.

On the physical plane, some of the key features are:

➤ Warmth aggravation

➤ Open air amelioration (especially anxiety)

➤ Motion amelioration

➤ Rich and fatty foods disagree

Menstrual disturbances or stomach ailments are a common companion of the chief complaints. Pulsatilla covers both Psora and Sycotic miasm.

[NOTE: In this case, the precursor was untraced. For details of the Journey of Disease refer to Chart no. 29]

▌█ REMEDY PRESCRIBED:

> ➤ Pulsatilla Nigricans 1M, 1 powder on 15/04/2017

▌█ FOLLOW-UPS:

30/05/2017

> ➤ Appetite improved.
> ➤ Vertigo on exertion, but was much better than before.
> ➤ Weakness had also improved markedly, where we could observe that she could sit comfortably, unlike the last time where she had to lie down.
> ➤ Breathlessness had also reduced, which was now only on ascending stairs.

▌█ PRESCRIPTION: Placebo

16/06/2017

> ➤ Last menstrual period - 10/06/2017.
> ➤ The flow was not heavy as before, no clots and bleeding lasted for 4 days.
> ➤ Had an episode of loose motion, with stool frequency of 4-5 times a day. But she had no weakness and breathlessness.

▌█ PRESCRIPTION: Placebo

08/07/2017

> ➤ Last menstrual period – 08/07/2017.
> ➤ The flow was very scanty as of now.
> ➤ Episode of urinary tract infection, increased urine frequency (5-6 times a day). Leucorrhoea since 8 days.
> ➤ Breathlessness and weakness was better.

▮▮ PRESCRIPTION: Pulsatilla Nigricans 1M,
1 powder was given.

26/07/2017

> ➤ Blackish discoloration in left axilla with itching. Ringworm infection. Was advised to avoid any application over the ringworm.
> ➤ Weakness and breathlessness much better.
> ➤ Had her menses, but the flow was very scanty and had bleeding only while passing urine.

▮▮ PRESCRIPTION: Placebo

08/08/2017

> ➤ Had menses, did not remember the date, but the flow was better this time.
> ➤ Weakness and breathlessness gradually improving.
> ➤ She was advised to get her Ultrasonography of the pelvis and complete blood count done for assessment.
> ➤ The Ultrasonography of the pelvis suggested the following :
>   • Fibroid showed no changes.
>   • CBC indicated improvement in the haemoglobin levels.

▮▮ PRESCRIPTION: Placebo

She showed gradual improvement since then.

ATOPIC DERMATITIS:
A WATCHFUL CHILD

DR. JAYESH DAVE

....

With the emergence of technology, the world has become a smaller place. In my goal of curing people of their ailments, technology has added a new dimension for doctors where we can treat even those patients for whom physical proximity for treatment is not possible. A similar kind of case appeared where I got an opportunity to undertake a virtual case from the United States (US) via Skype.

It was a case of Atopic Dermatitis, which revolved around a child of 5 months who had developed rashes all over the body. Her mother said, "On scratching, a yellow discharge oozes out of it." The treatment plan for it all over the US revolved around prescribing steroids which initially did help, but only for the rashes to reappear again. On revisiting the doctors, they asked the parents to perform all the allergic tests and avoid the potent allergens. Such a response from the doctors landed the parents in a state of discompose because they were looking for a permanent cure for their kid, and this really was not one. Seeking a permanent remedy for their child's sufferings, they contacted me through Skype.

On retrieving the medical history from her mother, we came to know the fact that when she was 1 month old, she used to bathe her with gram flour after which she had immediately developed rashes. When the child was born, there were no rashes. Rashes which had developed now were on the child's cheeks, forehead, arms, ankles and neck. Because of the rash, there was itching, which on scratching made the skin red. The child had also developed boils on the scalp, which appeared pustular.

We started to dig up a little more on the mother's pregnancy history, which was very vital in this case. On further interrogation, we found out that the mother had suffered 6 miscarriages before the birth of this child. Majority of the miscarriages happened during the second month (6th or 7th week, which could be due to any infection, for example: TORCH - Toxoplasmosis, Rubella, Cytomegalovirus, Herpes Simplex, Human Immunodeficiency virus). During the third miscarriage, she undertook an investigation in which an abnormal pair of chromosomes was detected on examination. During the final miscarriage, sudden bleeding had started, so Dilation and Curettage procedure was done, and the examination results came out to be normal.

On introspecting further, she recalled two incidents which occurred during her pregnancy which might have affected her. She recalled one incident where she had made a plan to go out with her husband but unfortunately on the very same day her husband encountered an accident and suffered a fracture. She had already suffered six miscarriages so she somehow consoled herself and decided not to stress much, as this would affect the health of the baby and at no cost was she ready to lose this baby due to stress.

She also told that she was grateful to her friends who helped her during this phase since her parents and in-laws were in India. She also revealed that there was a certain history between her in-laws and parents. Her in-laws and parents lacked the bonding which bothered her in terms of whom to call at the time of her delivery.

She also expressed that by nature she was very anxious and a pre-planner. In spite of all the problems between her in-laws and her parents, she always presented herself perfectly, as she did not want to hurt them. The constant bonding problem between her in-laws and parents irritated her and made her very anxious. This anxiety often made her skip her meals.

She was further asked to elaborate about her child's nature, which she described as restless. The baby could not sit idle and always moved her hands and legs; she was also very restless during her sleep. She further added that she loved nature and always smiled while looking at moving leaves and flowers. She liked polka dots and floral prints on clothes. Red colour attracted her. She was always curious to know about all the things and tried to catch all things. She preferred musical toys, especially *tabla*. Music helped her to sleep.

At public places too, she was very happy when people were around. She was very quiet, and if someone approached her for holding her, she happily and willingly went to them. She was moody at times but preferred attention and liked to be carried around. She was always watchful and always observed what her mother was doing.

On observing the baby on Skype, she was indeed a playful child, also restless during sleep which her mother had described. Mongolian marks were observed on buttocks, back and arm.

■ PHYSICAL GENERALS:

> Appetite: Good. Could not tolerate hunger
> Thirst: Not specified
> Likes: Not significant
> Dislikes: Not significant
> Stools: No complaints
> Urine: No complaints
> Perspiration: Moderate on scalp. Hair remained wet most of the time. Recurrent boils on scalp since 2 months
> Sleep: When born, did not sleep for much time – 30 minutes nap in general. Slept while feeding. Very active; even during sleep restlessness was marked. Eyes were closed but she was moving.
> Thermals: Hot patient. Palms were always warm, moist and sweaty

▮▮ Sensitivity

- ➤ Sun: Not significant
- ➤ Noise: Startled if something came suddenly. Enjoyed going out in public gatherings. No problem with noise.
- ➤ Light: Not significant.
- ➤ Taste: Not significant.

▮▮ SUMMARY OF THE CASE

The following case lays down a brief summary about a child who was suffering from skin rashes. In order to find a possible remedy for this case, a detailed case history of the mother was undertaken. In this case, the child's mother had a recurrent history of 6 miscarriages especially during the second month of every pregnancy. She conceived this child during her seventh pregnancy; she recalled and described herself to be in a very anxious state of mind. She was often concerned about her husband but at the same time she was aware of the fact that she should not undergo a miscarriage due to the stress.

The continuous history of repeated miscarriage indicated that the child's mother must be suffering from some infection, most probably TORCH, which the child must have encountered in the womb, as there were no clear outward manifestations. It was also brought to our notice that immediately after birth, the child had suffered from jaundice. For it, she was given light therapy in higher intermediate zone and as child's vitality was not affected much, the jaundice was resolved.

When she was 1 month old, skin eruptions flared up after applying gram flour, which was an exciter due to which rashes appeared. The rashes were later diagnosed as Atopic Dermatitis. Previously, it was misdiagnosed as Seborrheic Dermatitis, Cradle Cap, Urticaria and so on.

Atopic Dermatitis is a skin condition, which is characterised by skin dryness with fissures and has a high risk of Eczema due to functional impairment in the epidermal structural protein (Filagarin protein), which causes disturbance in the skin barrier. This impairment is caused due to the combined effect of environmental and immune disturbances, thus leading to Atopy. In this case, the immune system of the child got affected due to mother's infection during pregnancy and got accelerated due to causes like gram flour and the emotional state of mother during that period.

This child was described as a restless baby, who could not sit idle and had to continuously move. She was also described as restless even during her sleep. By nature, she was a happy child who was also an extrovert. She loved nature and was fond of colours. She was a very alert and watchful child.

▎▎ Rubrics considered were:

> ➤ Mind; AILMENTS from anticipation, foreboding, presentiment (Derived from mother's history during pregnancy)

▎▎ Rubrics based on Observation:

> ➤ Mind; TOSSING about General sleep, during
> ➤ Mind; EXTROVERTED
> ➤ Mind; WATCHFULNESS

Two remedies bearing resemblance with the case were Sulphur and Phosphorus due to their common facets of watchfulness and being extroverted. However, the child did not portray fear, which forms an important aspect of Phosphorus. Moreover, the child being thermally hot, we prescribed Sulphur.

[NOTE: In this case, the precursor was untraced. For details of the Journey of Disease refer to Chart no. 27]

▌▌ REMEDY PRESCRIBED:

> ➤ Sulphur 200, 1 powder was given on 6/10/2017

▌▌ FOLLOW-UPS:

30/10/2017

> ➤ Rashes came and went on their own, that too on previous scars only.
> ➤ Also yesterday had developed boils after oiling of the body, but they got settled on washing the parts.
> ➤ Two episodes of cold and cough, but she required no treatment, as it settled gradually on its own.
> ➤ Also, she was advised to stop applying gram flour and milk on the skin.

▌▌ PRESCRIPTION: Placebo

13/01/2018

> ➤ On eating *dosa* (fermented food), allergic rashes had developed
> ➤ The mother mentioned that she had applied gram flour to the baby intermittently, but this time the baby did not get eruptions like previously.

▌▌ PRESCRIPTION: Placebo

04/04/2018

> ➤ No redness, no allergic episodes. Even if eruptions came, they disappeared on their own within a few minutes.
> ➤ Heat boils over the neck during summers.
> ➤ Her mother had now started feeding her egg yolk and chicken, but they did not cause any problem to the baby.
> ➤ Sleep was disturbed; she got up in between then slept again after a while. Restlessness during sleep was better than before.

▮▮ PRESCRIPTION: Placebo

06/10/2018

> ➢ She developed rashes behind the knees
> ➢ Sleep was better. Now no restlessness during sleep
> ➢ Started with egg white but no complaints
> ➢ Active, impatient child. Someone had to be there with her

▮▮ PRESCRIPTION: Placebo

Patient was still under treatment and child was doing well. She was able to eat non-vegetarian food without any allergy. Rash behind knee was gradually improving although she itched a lot. She had been on placebo since then.

HIDRADENITIS SUPPURATIVA:
IF I AM NOT APPRECIATED, I GET HURT

DR. LAI SANGOI

In the year 2017, an adolescent girl visited my clinic. Before coming to the clinic, she had called up to know whether a condition 'Hidradenitis Suppurativa' could be treated with Homoeopathy. Unaware of the disease, I told her to come to my clinic and show me the reports and her medical file. On further studies, I came to know that Hidradenitis Suppurativa is a rare skin disorder, a long-term skin disease characterised by occurrence of inflamed and swollen lumps. These are typically painful and break open releasing fluid or pus. Areas commonly affected are arm pits, below the breast and groin region. Self-consciousness and depression may result during the course of treatment, as it is incurable according to the modern medicine.

The following day, the patient was accompanied by her mother. Their faces portrayed sheer worry and discomfort. The reason for their worry was that they had done a lot of treatment for this ailment, but there were no signs of relief even after continuous and varied medications.

Ongoing through the patient's file, her dermatologist had diagnosed her with Hidradenitis Suppurativa along with Comedonal Acne. This was a great opportunity for me, as people always feel that complex or incurable diseases cannot be cured by Homoeopathy. As stated by Dr. Hahnemann in *The Chronic Diseases*, "Treatment by allopathic physicians hitherto merely serves to increase the distress from this kind of disease. If the patient kept on taking the crude medicines and harmful local application, instead of the former sufferings, there would appear a worse state-nameless disease caused by medicine, far worse and more incurable than the original natural one."

Being a firm believer of my science, I knew that we would be able to treat her more rationally if we understood the individual as a whole and not just the particular disease.

Having a distressing experience with allopathic treatment, they were hopeful about homoeopathic treatment. On enquiring as to what exactly were the complaints and how they began, the duo narrated the following:

Multiple pustular eruptions around the vaginal region on both sides. Eruptions aggravating during onset of menses. Burning pain, aggravation by slightest touch – screams due to pain. She further added that the eruptions were very painful, and she was not able to bear them. She was not able to sit and could not even wear sanitary pads because of the discomfort it caused.

"The pain makes me angry," she said. "I get irritated when it pains. When my mother used to apply ointment, it would burn like hell, and I kept on shouting and weeping and would also kick my mother. I would not pass urine frequently, as it would burn. Doctor had told us that after applying ointment, cracks would form, and it will take time to heal. The same thing happened, and I had deep cracks and also bleeding."

Onset, Duration and Progress: Slight itching over vaginal area before menarche; was treated with local ointments. After her first menses, there appeared few eruptions around the vaginal area. She said that the eruptions started as small ones and gradually increased in size. Her General Physician prescribed some medicines but nothing helped, and eruptions would recur with more pains and distress.

Further, the mother expressed her concern about her daughter's menses, saying that they had been irregular since menarche. They were always delayed and flow once started would be scanty, red and would last for 10-15 days. Also, she had acne on her face, with some painful pustular boils. The eruptions were better after applying local ointments.

The girl was more bothered about her weight, which she started gaining after 7th grade. She said, "Initially I was very fair and good looking, but now have put on a lot of weight, which I don't like at all."

She generally looked down, and her voice had a low tone while speaking.

She further narrated, "I want to look pretty and thin. I love wearing nice clothes and shorts. But lately due to my weight, I am not able to wear them. Others can wear, and I cannot. I feel bad when I see others looking prettier. This makes me angry, as my friends have started teasing me. I do not like people judging me; how can they judge me on my weight and looks (she was weeping while narrating this)? My friends call me fat. Although I do not react, I feel angry from within."

Question asked: *"What has affected you the most? Why are you weeping so much?"*

There was pin-drop silence and no response at all, which made me send her mother out. Still she seemed reluctant to answer my questions. This led me to explain to her importance of mental faculty in the harmonious functioning of the body. Her weeping became more intense, she shrugged her shoulders, and her fist was tightly closed. She finally started detailing about a dispute she had with a friend when she was in 9th grade. She said, "There was a misunderstanding between me and my best friend, and our friendship broke. My friend bitched about me, and that created a misunderstanding. I was wrongly blamed for no fault of mine, and so my friends started avoiding me. I felt very bad about it. That incidence still hurts me because we had a good group, and I was not a part of it anymore. They would avoid me when I approached them. I felt lonely during that time. This was a tough phase of my life. I wanted my friends to trust me, but none of them did. I could not focus on my studies; I was completely shattered."

She was silent after narrating the above incident but could still not control her tears.

Question asked – "*How are you as a person?*"

She said, "I always liked being in a joint family because I like people being around me. I am an emotional person, and I get hurt easily. If someone talks rudely to me, it affects me."

Her mother narrated further that since childhood she had been emotional. "She feels that I always take the side of her younger brother and shout at her." Her mother continued saying that she was an aggressive child and got irritated by small things. Once angry, she locked the door and stayed alone. She was very anxious especially before her exams; she always wept a day before exams thinking about what would happen.

"She was a bright student till the 6th grade, but after that her marks have been consistently low, which is not the case with my younger one. He is bright and smart." To this, she immediately reacted, "I was also smart when I was of his age."

Hobbies: "I love dancing, but in our school, teachers show a lot of partiality. They always prefer other students. I feel bad that because of my weight my teachers are not selecting me. I am always chosen second, and it hurts me very much."

PHYSICAL GENERALS

- ➤ Appearance: Obesity with acne on face
- ➤ Appetite: She was a foodie and loved eating junk food
- ➤ Thermals: Hot patient
- ➤ Thirst: Thirsty
- ➤ Dreams: At times, she got frightful dreams and slept beside her mother
- ➤ Fear: Fear of the dark; even at this age she did not go to the washroom alone at night, or she would keep the door open. She said, "I cannot stay alone in the dark, I get scared." Her mother said, "The younger one is bolder than her."

██ ANALYSIS OF THE CASE:

Homoeopathy is not meant to treat cold and cough. The so-called incurable diseases termed by modern medicine can be completely cured by our sweet medicines in the most harmless way.

The child was very sensitive especially to the situation that happened in 9th grade, where her friends did not trust her and left her. She felt lonely after that situation, and now she did not trust anyone easily.

Her weight was affecting her, and she felt jealous when others were looking good or wearing good clothes compared to her. Similar jealousy was seen in school where teachers preferred others to her. She was too concerned about what people said about her or their opinion. Fear of the dark was also marked.

At the physical level, she was extremely sensitive to pain and could not bear it; she has a tendency for pustular boils and obesity. She was lazy as claimed by her mother and avoided physical exertion.

> Weight: 83 kg

██ Rubrics considered were:

> Mind; FORSAKEN feeling
> Mind; JEALOUSY General
> Generals; SENSITIVENESS pain to
> Mind; FEAR dark

[NOTE: In this case, the precursor was untraced. For details of the Journey of Disease refer to Chart no. 24]

██ REMEDY PRESCRIBED:

> Calcarea Sulphurica 200, 1 powder given on 13/07/2017

▮▮ FOLLOW-UPS:

19/07/2017

> ➤ Ultrasonography of abdomen and pelvis indicated Grade 1 Fatty liver.
> ➤ No new eruptions.
> ➤ Eruptions which were present earlier had now subsided.
> ➤ Pain was severe when she had come for consultation; now it was better.
> ➤ Mentally also, her anger had reduced now.

▮▮ PRESCRIPTION: Placebo

28/07/2017

> ➤ Eruptions had subsided compared to before
> ➤ She complained of sneezing in between for 2 days. Otherwise, overall, she was better
> ➤ She had recently started with guitar classes. She was looking much happier and more positive than before. She said, "Now what my friends think of me does not affect me." Weight – 78 kg

▮▮ PRESCRIPTION: Placebo

16/1/2018

> ➤ Eruptions had completely disappeared, no pain, no rashes
> ➤ Menses had been regular since the past three months
> ➤ Mild eruptions (acne) on the forehead
> ➤ Her weight was also reducing and she felt more energetic than before. "I am so relaxed because the terrible pain of eruptions has gone."

▌▐ PRESCRIPTION: Placebo

APPRECIATE MY STORY: CALCAREA SULPHURICA

"I am a girl who loves to get attention, but due to my weight I am not looking good. Please don't judge me according to my weight; I am a very sensitive girl, and rudeness and criticism affects me too much. Appreciate me for my good skills; when you can appreciate others then why not me? Mom, I don't like it when you compare me with others. I know my inabilities, and I get jealous when I see others getting more attention or getting ahead of me. I feel that I am not being valued and not being given the desired importance. Facing the public is like a real task for me, and I feel shy when I am with strangers or new people. I will excel in life if you support me, mom. Doing things alone is a task for me. Before doing new things or before exams I get very tense and have constant thoughts about whether I will do well or not; my confidence is low, and many times I have black outs before exams. Keep boosting me, so my confidence will boost up. If I am neglected then I will be deeply hurt and go into my shell, and sadness will prevail. I hate exertion and like luxuries of life. People generally call me lazy, and I do accept it. This is me, in short. Do appreciate my story, for as you know, if I am not valued, I will lament about it."

CASE 8

FOCAL CYSTIC ENCEPHALOMALACIA: AN ILL-HUMOURED CHILD

DR. VASANTH DHARMARAJ

In the month of March 2016, a physiotherapist friend of mine referred a patient, a baby aged 18 months, who was diagnosed as Chronic Left Middle Cerebral Artery Infarct with Focal Cystic Encephalomalacia and presented with complaints of paresis of the right arm, difficulty in standing and inability to walk. Moreover, whenever the parents made an attempt to make him walk, he had a disturbed gait. On talking with the parents, it was likely that they had no clear idea about what was going on with their kid. They belonged to an illiterate family with poor medical awareness and were taken aback by the present state of their little one.

They seemed to be extremely worried and had given up after trying every possible expert on the ailment that their child suffered from. On asking as to what were his present complaints, the parents narrated that he could not hold things with his hands, and that if it had to be done, he would end up using only his left hand. He could not stand. It felt as if he had no strength to do so. On attempting to walk, he always dragged his left leg and kept stumbling whereas the right leg was absolutely normal. The mother added, "We have also started him with calcium and vitamin supplements so that it aids him with all this. He gets too exhausted after exercising, and this has been since the time his physiotherapy began. This is so extreme that he goes off to sleep there itself."

Further interrogation also revealed that he had delayed global milestones. Now the current state of his made it difficult for him to even sit on his own; he could not walk, and the parents were anticipating that their child would become handicapped.

On further asking as to when these changes had been first observed, the parents could trace all of this back to when their child was 6 months old. That was when all of it started. They first noticed his right hand became rigid and his fist always used to remain closed. And the further changes then followed.

On probing the child's birth history, it was discovered that the baby weighed 3.5 kilograms when delivered and was delivered through a caesarean, had not cried after birth and had aspirated meconium, which had resulted into Congenital Pneumonia with stage 2 HIE (Hypoxic Ischemic Encephalopathy) at the time of birth. The doctors had no hope and asked for an immediate shift to the Neonatal Intensive Care Unit. He had to be kept on ventilation, and this was his state for almost a month. On asking why a caesarean was performed, she mentioned that she had high blood pressure during her first pregnancy; so to avoid any damage to the kid, a planned caesarean was done.

Further describing his state of health since birth, the mother seemed to be extremely anxious as she said that her kid always had some or the other health issue since the very beginning. Every time the weather changed or he had the slightest of cold things, he would suffer from a respiratory infection with nose block, severe coryza and cough with white to greenish expectoration. "He is so sensitive that we cannot feed him sour, oily, spicy or cold things. He has difficulty in breathing during the episode, and this happens at least once a month. This is accompanied with fever. He has cough with expectoration which is variable, and is sticky white. His cough gets so severe that he ends up vomiting, and he throws out everything that he eats. Even the change in water when we visit our native makes him sick. He gets too disturbed when he is not well. He becomes irritable and keeps nagging continuously. Also stops having any food. He just wants someone to carry him."

On further asking her to elaborate the kid's nature, she described that he was extremely mischievous but he had no strength, due to which he got tired easily. "He will not put in efforts to do things by himself, he will ask me or someone to get things for him. He is also very restless. He mixes easily with everyone but when with new people he takes time. He gets angry if you do not listen to him. And when angry, he would throw things around. He would bang his head and hit people around."

"For instance, if his cousin who is younger than him tries getting close and he does not like it, then he will bite her and will also snatch her hair. He will always try to protect himself. He will never share his belongings. If the other children in the family take any of his toys, he will hit them with his legs. If anyone teases him, he does not take it and hits the person and starts screaming. He would sometimes share, but he gets offended if anyone snatches something from his hand. If you go close to him, touch him when he does not want you to, he will spit on the opposite person. He will call out the names of the elderly people in the family. But when his grandmother scolds him, he gets scared and hides behind. He does this also when you say something repeatedly."

"Both he and his elder brother are similar; they do not get scared of anything. But he is very stubborn. As in, if he wants something and we do not give it, he will get irritated. If you offer it later, he won't take it then. Initially, he will keep demanding and throw temper tantrums. He is not fearful otherwise, but he is scared of animals. Even if a cat passes by, he will get scared and move away. All kind of animals scare him."

"He gets annoyed if anyone disturbs him when he is busy doing something. Even our neighbours—he doesn't like it when they kiss him, even out of love. He is moody. He enjoys watching cartoons, colourful things. He loves dancing and loud music. Though his body is not fit for it, he tries dancing in his own way."

"Also, the doctor had mentioned an abnormality which we never realised until we saw changes in him when he was 6 months old. We visited many experts for his illness but all was in vain. We were told that the only solution we had for him was physiotherapy; that too it would only be compensation, for no total cure is assured." While describing all this, the father of the child mentioned something which was striking and had to be investigated further. He said the gynaecologist they consulted throughout the pregnancy had already warned them of the harm of continuing the pregnancy, as there was a chance of delivering an abnormal baby. This was told in the first trimester itself when they had got her ultrasonography done. In spite of all this, they decided to continue the pregnancy, and she was advised complete bed rest throughout.

This indicated that the outcome now faced by the kid was a reflection of some gross reason back then during her pregnancy, which was an important aspect to be known.

On asking the mother to describe her state of health during the nine months, she just went on with her endless stuff which suggested that she had a hard time while she was pregnant. She narrated, "I was troubled by the nausea and vomiting, which was not relieved by any treatment. And during the first three months, I had recurrent episodes of severe urinary tract infection. I had burning micturition right from the first month. This was added with mental stress, which took a toll on me. I used to be very frustrated. The doctor had advised me complete bed rest, but the state was total opposite; my elder son was just one and a half years old, and I had to work all day. Our family had also got separated, which increased my stress. There was a constant nagging in the house. I used to get irritated due to all this. Even if I woke up late on any of the mornings, I had to face so many questions. They made me get up in the middle of my sleep. I was not able to work due to the breathing complaint. I had constant anxiety and palpitations, which made it worse. They used to trouble me a lot, and I had no option other than to work all day from early morning till late night. I was worried all nine months about my child. I used to keep on thinking if my baby would be fine. I just had faith in God. I was very frustrated, as things were not getting well, and I had to work on an empty stomach."

"Above all, I could never answer back. My parents were everything for me. My family did not pay attention to my health then, and now they blame me for everything saying that I did not exercise and take proper rest. My parents stayed far away hence I could not go to their place. I had become extremely angry, and it all came out on my husband. My brother-in-law kept nagging. I was continuously worried, as it was too early that I had conceived, and I could not nurture my other kid as well. This kept bothering my mind."

"Finally, I went to my brother's place in the ninth month, even after the doctor asked me not to travel. There was no peace of mind here. I was ready to work, but I wanted no fights. This kept constantly piling up the anger within me all throughout the pregnancy."

▮▮ PHYSICAL GENERALS:

> Appetite: Good. Could tolerate hunger
> Likes: Not significant
> Dislikes: Not significant
> Thirst: He did not drink much water. Thirstless
> Urine: No complaints
> Stool: Passed stools twice a day. Offensive stools
> Perspiration: Moderate. More over scalp
> Sleep: Refreshing
> Thermals: Hot patient

▮▮ SUMMARY OF THE CASE

The year 2016 provided me a great teaching from the encounter of a jumbled-up case of Focal Cystic Encephalomalacia and recurrent respiratory tract infection, where no head and tail of the inception of the disease was clear. The child was presented with paresis of the right hand and left leg. In this maze of symptoms, I first thought of searching for the cause of his ailments. I came across an MRI report of the child at 11 months, which displayed Chronic Left Middle Cerebral Artery Infarct. This was the indication of an old assault to the brain tissue.

On trying to trace still rearward, the discharge summary of the kid indicated evidence of HIE Stage 2 (Hypoxic Ischaemic Encephalopathy) with meconium-stained amniotic fluid. This suggested an oxygen-deprived state of the brain cells whose likely reflection was the infarct.

Having not yet discovered the cause of the foetal stress, I decided to explore the pregnancy history. An important finding was that the mother continuously suffered from Urinary Tract Infection without any vaginal discharge during the first trimester of her pregnancy.

Reading about it, I astonishingly found that studies suggest that ascending Urinary Tract Infections (UTI) in pregnant mothers can lead to damage to the foetal brain cells or premature labour. Moreover, these congenital foetal infections from the mother are also potent in damaging the foetal brain cells. This eventuates by the activation of inflammatory cascade pathways, anaerobic reactions and hypoxia, which leads to cell death and necrosis. Thus, we could correlate the probable reason for the gynaecologist advising termination of pregnancy during the 1st trimester.

Thus, we could rightly infer that the persistent UTI in mother during the 1st trimester of pregnancy led to the chronicity in the child. The organisms responsible for producing UTI without vaginal discharge during pregnancy are Escherichia Coli, Group B Streptococcus, Staphylococcus, Virus and Fungus. These agents can enter the body by multiple routes other than sexual. Thus, this case can be classified as a miasmatic disease of non-venereal origin, i.e., Psora (For details of the Journey of Disease refer to Chart no. 25).

The Pneumonia that the child contracted soon after birth was a possible opportunistic infection, which added to the chronicity already started in the body.

The mother also mentioned her emotion of anger that prevailed all through her pregnancy. This was triggered by incessant nagging by her in-laws. Although she was advised complete bed rest all through her pregnancy, she was made to work round the clock, which further evoked anger. In spite of being breathless, she would complete all the chores without any retaliation. When furious with anger, it was expressed only on her husband.

This continuous anger served as an exciting cause, which added fuel to the fire and led to the passage of meconium by the baby in-utero.

In my clinical observation, I came to acknowledge that the baby principally acquires and reflects the very same or the exact opposite emotion that the mother eminently feels all through her pregnancy. In this case as well, the child was an angry kid, bearing similitude with his mother. He was very sensitive to being forced and always retorted to it. His expression was always seen in the form of anger, which was demonstrated in a timid way by either throwing things away, banging his head, biting and spitting on his known people.

One more aspect which revealed the child's haughtily-angry behaviour was that he expressed irritability on being offered something later, which was not given when he first asked for it. Another segment of his behaviour was his fear of animals. One more notable facet was his desire to be carried whenever he was unwell.

▌ Rubrics considered were:

> ➤ Generals; SIDE crosswise left lower and right upper
> ➤ Mind; Ailments from anger, vexation
> ➤ Mind; Striking general
> ➤ Mind; Fear animals of

Two remedies which came in close proximity were Platina and Lycopodium Clavatum. Platina could be ruled out, as Platina children are averse to be carried and desire to be alone; unlike Lycopodium children who do not leave their mother, as they fear being alone and are hesitant to meet new people.

This case was a perfect picture of a timid but angry Lycopodium child. My experience with Lycopodium children has taught me about their contrary exhibition, either as a docile child or a very disobedient one, but the emotion of anger is a common companion.

In the case of disobedient children, it is usually seen that they express their anger on their parents to the extent of abusing and insulting them. An incident that is strongly embossed in my mind is of a child I met in a camp who came to seek consultation. He sat on his father's lap. One of the assistants snatched something from the child's hand. To this he reacted in a very shocking manner by slapping his father in front of everyone. This vividly displayed his anger as well as his timidity.

It is also observed that Lycopodium children when unwell can be highly peevish and ill-humoured where they can go to the extent of striking their known people.

On the other hand, a complete different picture of Lycopodium is seen where although anger prevails, it is subdued and they are extremely obedient, meek and mild. This is mostly seen in cases where there is a history of strict parenting. These children are very conscientious about their studies and its incompletion brings on anxiety. This anxiety is also seen before their results.

In my years of clinical practice, I have mostly observed Lycopodium children holding their mother's hand or their clothes while entering the physician's cabin, which is mostly due to the fear of facing new people.

■■ REMEDY PRESCRIBED:

➤ Lycopodium Clavatum 200, 1 powder on 22/03/2016
➤ Physiotherapy to be continued as an auxiliary mode.

■■ FOLLOW-UPS:

30/05/2016
➤ There was no episode of cold and cough in the past 2 months.
➤ Had now started lifting his right hand; movements improved. But still could not hold things with right hand.
➤ Also, could stand for a while without falling.
➤ Speech had improved.

▌▐ PRESCRIPTION: Placebo

09/08/2016

> ➤ Overall, the child was improving; he had no episode of respiratory infection since March 2016.
> ➤ Used both his hands well, but still could not hold things with right hand though he tried to do so.
> ➤ Now walked with the help of a walker but could not stand for a long time as he did in the first month after medicine.

▌▐ PRESCRIPTION: Placebo

12/10/2016

> ➤ His mother said, "He is better, but the improvement in last 2 months is the same. No further improvement is seen; he does not stand, though he tries."
> ➤ No episode of cold and cough.

▌▐ PRESCRIPTION: Lycopodium Clavatum200, 1 powder was repeated.

25/03/2017

> ➤ The child was still not able to hold things with his right hand. But the movements of the hand had improved. Opened the fist, which he initially kept closed, but did not have a grip to hold with it.
> ➤ He could now speak well, and could understand and comprehend things in a better way.
> ➤ Had an episode of cold, cough after he had ice cream, had difficulty in breathing for a while, but that did not continue and settled without any interference. Also, he did not have a greenish discharge from the throat during this episode.

➤ He could sit folding his legs, and his strength in the legs had improved, he would now touch the medial aspect of his left leg (foot) to the ground when he walked.

▮▮ PRESCRIPTION: Placebo

After a continuous treatment of 2 years, the child had gradually improved. He had now started walking without any support. Also, he now kicked a ball and gait had improved. The movement and grip of the right hand improved, though the strength was still less than the left hand.

A single dose of Lycopodium 200 was repeated when he had an episode of worms. There was also some tightness of the right hand since sometime in the month of November 2017. He had episodes of cold, cough for a few times, but this time without any fever or breathlessness.

He showed gradual improvement since then.

ICHTHYOSIS: THE CONCURRENCE OF FICTIONAL TERROR AND FISHY SKIN

DR. RAJAN DUBEY & DR. HARSHITA VORA

....

A 15-month-old baby diagnosed with Ichthyosis since birth was carried by her mother to us in the month of January 2012. She complained that the baby got severe redness and itching of skin during summer, so much so that she got completely red from top to bottom, including her eyelids. She had parched skin because of which she could not even close her eyelids completely.

On enquiring how exactly the symptoms were noticed, her mother explained that the situation was much better now, as they frequently applied oil to maintain the moisture of the skin. Immediately after her birth, she could notice dryness and scaling every time she bathed her and thought it was a normal dryness of skin. 10-15 days later, it started worsening and her skin soon started appearing like plastic. It was only then that they consulted a doctor for their daughter, who was then diagnosed with this condition.

Further, she narrated about her daughter's complaint by saying, "She develops severe dryness during summer. She has to be bathed 4-5 times with water. If she is exposed to the sun for even 5 minutes then she immediately turns red. Usually, I bathe her once in 10-15 days during cold weather and rainy season, as she immediately develops cold to the extent that she suffers from Pneumonia. Even when we bathe her once in 10 days she starts with cold, cough and wheezing. There is intense itching; she keeps on scratching and cries until water or oil is applied. Also, I observed this one unusual thing: until she is wearing her clothes there is no itching."

We could observe thick scab formation over the scalp of the baby. On asking more about it to her mother, she mentioned that they had to apply oil for 3-4 hours after which the scabs would fall off while combing her hair.

As the complaint had started ever since birth, we had to elucidate the mother's history during pregnancy. On doing so, we received the following details:

Recollecting her phase of pregnancy, she proclaimed about her complaints during that period. "I had chronic leucorrhoea which used to be thick, white and profuse accompanied with itching in the vaginal area. I had this since 12 years, but this persisted all throughout my pregnancy. I also had vomiting during my pregnancy. I was not able to even tolerate the sight of food, and this continued even after the delivery of my baby. This had been my state during all the three pregnancies. I had taken treatment in the initial months for piles. I had 3-4 episodes of bleeding per rectum which settled after the medication."

"During the initial days of the 8th month, I had sudden pain. When I consulted my gynaecologist for the pain, it was discovered that due to polyhydramnios, the external cervical os had opened that eventually led to premature birth. Also, the delivered baby was in the footling breech presentation. Before the 8th month, everything seemed normal as per the sonography reports."

She suddenly seemed to become emotional while she unexpectedly started mentioning her previous abortion history, where due to her health issues, the doctor had advised her to terminate the pregnancy. She said, "There was a possibility of threat to me or my baby, and hence I had to abort it against my will. But this kept haunting me ever since then. I used to feel I will be punished for this sin even after my death. This fear which I had developed since then is still affecting me till date. I again conceived within 3-4 months after this abortion, which was an unwanted one. I continuously had this thought in my mind that I should have not committed the sin of aborting that baby. I also had a fear that nothing should go wrong during this delivery and even if it did, I would give birth to this child. I won't be repeating that mistake again."

She was further asked to elaborate the child's nature, to which she described by saying, "My baby is a playful child. She mixes easily with people around. She starts dancing when she hears music. I have observed she fears strangers especially those who have a long beard. She cannot stay alone and wants people around her. But you just sit beside her, don't touch or carry her. If her favourite thing is snatched by someone she does not like it; if it is with someone she will snatch it back. If someone puts her on their lap, she starts crying. She gets happy when she sees cats; she will call out my name and tell me about it. She gets excited when she sees animals. She is very smart for her age. When she observes me making dough she too would try doing that. Also when I rinse the utensils she will offer soap to me. She will help me clean the vegetables."

"She is an observant child. If you give her a book, she would start reading and scribbling. She would mimic things by observing them. If she is crying while I am feeding her, she stops crying and has the milk if I turn on the radio. None of the things is taught to her. She likes to apply *mehendi*. First thing she would want me to do is comb her hair. To mention an incident, when I took her yesterday to a shop, she was not allowing me to pay until I bought her a biscuit, which she demanded."

On observation: She was trying to talk to her mother and called her continuously during case-taking. She cried twice during case-taking, but she stopped crying after weaning.

■ PHYSICAL GENERALS:

> Appetite: She could tolerate hunger. She preferred milk during sleep especially at night. Her mother said if her sleep was disrupted at night and if she did not see her mother around, she cried aloud. So to make her quiet she had to be breastfed.

> Aversion: Did not like sweets at all. She would spit it out. Also did not like bitter & spicy taste.

> Thirst: She drank water while eating food. If she saw her parents drinking it, she will ask for it. She would never drink milk through artificial nipple; she would take it in a spoon.

> Stool: No complaints

> Urine: No complaints

> Perspiration: Occasionally on the tip of the nose. Otherwise did not perspire.

> Sleep: Refreshing; she got up if there was a noise of utensils.

> Thermals: Hot patient. She could not tolerate heat. She did not like covering her face with a blanket during sleep. She would remove it from the face.

■ SUMMARY OF THE CASE

This here is a case of Ichthyosis, which is a rare genetic disorder. Ichthyosis comes from a Greek word *'ichthys'* that literally means 'fish' – since dry, scaly skin (thick or thin) is the defining feature of all forms of Ichthyosis. It can be due to genetic mutation or acquired during life. There occurs a genetic mutation whereby the protein responsible to protect the skin and keep it moist, gets affected.

In this case, the child's mother had a longstanding history of leucorrhoea, which even persisted throughout the pregnancy. This served as a precursor which led to the genetic mutation in the child in the form of Ichthyosis. Having already known that the causes of leucorrhoea are:

1. Physiological – due to oestrogenic stimulation, or
2. Due to infection – bacterial or parasitic like Chlamydia or Trichomonas

Supporting our speculation, a research at the Max Planck Institute for Infection Biology (Germany) revealed that sexually-transmitted diseases can cause mutation in the host DNA by overriding the normal mechanism.

I have come to realise that in paediatric cases, the pregnancy history holds significance as long as the disease exists in its primitive stage. Once the disease changes its form and emerges with a different name, the pregnancy history tends to lose its profundity.

Once the precursor establishes chronicity in the body, the exciting factors play a mere role of budding up the disease. On retrieving the mother's pregnancy history, it was evident that she was in a state of constant anxiety about having committed a sin by aborting her former child, and she felt she would be punished for the same even in her after life. There was a sustained piling up of this emotion throughout her pregnancy.

Numerous studies have confirmed that the neurotransmitters released by the pregnant mother's body in response to anxiety, stress or fear are transported into the womb and affect the unborn baby.

In the above mentioned case, we could perceive that the mother's state throughout the pregnancy which evidently highlighted the emotion of 'fear of salvation' was also noticed in the child who became fearful whenever she came across people with strange faces. Thus, we could infer that the fear in both the mother and the child held close resemblance by virtue of being fictitious.

As a compensation for her fear, the child portrayed herself as a very playful and extroverted child. Other attributes of her behaviour showed her love for animals, fear of being alone and an aversion to being touched or carried.

▌ Rubrics considered were:

> ➤ Generals; FOOD and drinks sweets aversion
> ➤ Generals; SUN from exposure to agg. or ailments from
> ➤ Skin; ERUPTIONS scaly ichthyosis
> ➤ Skin; ITCHING undressing agg.

In my practical experience, I have come to acknowledge that a firm foundation is majorly provided by the generals and particulars thus enabling us to comprehend the case distinctly. The remedy was finally selected taking into consideration the mother's pregnancy history and the child's history. On repertorisation, the three remedies that came closer were Sulphur, Medorrhinum and Pulsatilla Nigricans. Pulsatilla children not only crave love but are also very affectionate, and they are fond of being caressed. Thus, Pulsatilla was ruled out.

The major crux of the case was the aspect of fear, which was evidently seen in both the mother and the child. Bearing this in mind, the remedy that was apparently similar was Medorrhinum as 'Obscure Fear' comprises a salient feature of this remedy. This non-descript fear is so much that they constantly fret that something disagreeable would happen. This sustained emotion of fear gives rise to an enormous degree of anticipation in them, where they start predicting events. Their forecast also comes to life but majorly for unpleasant occurrences. A ceaseless feeling of having done an unpardonable offence persists and the sequel is a state of dilemma – 'Will I attain Moksha?' 'Will I be sent to heaven or hell?'

Medorrhinum patients are much occupied with their imaginary fears like fear of misfortune, hearing voices, being pursued, etc. This fear keeps them so absorbed that over the time, their concentration becomes difficult and memory becomes dull, which is appreciated when they lose track or are unable to complete a conversation as they forget what they intend to say. This memory dullness is so overpowering that they sometimes even forget their own name and on being questioned, they tend to repeat the same. They always have a rush of ideas but cannot complete it and hence they procrastinate.

Other facets of Medorrhinum include:
- Extreme nervousness which makes them hurried.
- Weeping while narrating their symptoms, which is a prominent feature.
- Over sensitiveness to criticism and contradiction.

I have observed two contrasting states of Medorrhinum:

One where they appear to be oversensitive, nervous, impulsive, abrupt, egoistic and cruel and on the other hand they are sad, tearful, fearful, sympathetic and lack confidence.

Some of the key attributes of Medorrhinum are:

> Desire open air

> Biting nails

> Lying on abdomen

One more remedy coming close was Sulphur, but disposition-wise they are very happy-go-lucky and cheerful people. Sulphur was ruled out because of the higher degree of fear and anxiety about salvation, which was seen in our patient. Sulphur and Medorrhinum share a common aspect of procrastination. Medorrhinum patients postpone things out of memory weakness and a fear of taking up responsibilities, whereas a Sulphur patient would postpone things merely due to his frivolous nature.

This case approached me in the year of 2012, while I was still researching on miasms. However, recently a telephonic conversation with the patient's mother revealed that she was till date suffering from leucorrhoea. This confirmed my speculation that the leucorrhoea was sexually transmitted. Thus, Medorrhinum worked miraculously in this incurable case, as it was a miasmatic disease of venereal origin (For details of the Journey of Disease refer to Chart no. 17).

▌▌ REMEDY PRESCRIBED:

> Medorrhinum 200, 1 powder on 02/01/2012

▌▌ FOLLOW-UPS:

> ➤ The family shifted to Pune and thus the follow-up was maintained on call with a simultaneous observation by a colleague over there who had referred the case to me.
> ➤ In recent follow-up conversation with her father, he mentioned that she was much better and improving gradually. The scaling of skin and dryness was better. She could now move her neck, which was restricted due to extreme dryness and scaling.
> ➤ No repetition was done after the first dose, and they were advised to apply oil over the skin to avoid discomfort to the child.

SYSTEMIC LUPUS ERYTHEMATOSUS: AN EDUCATOR DREADING DISGRACE

DR. RAJAN DUBEY & DR. SNEHA SHARMA

....

After having consulted numerous well-known physicians for her illness and having developed the dread of living a life being dependent on immunosuppressants, a 32-year-old female came to visit us in the summer of 2016. Being a teacher by profession, she was very well acquainted with the adverse effects of the steroids, which she was prescribed for her disease diagnosed as Systematic Lupus Erythematosus, an auto-immune condition. She presented herself to us in a state of extreme pain, which made it difficult for her to even get up from the chair.

Her clinical reports also suggested a positive Antinuclear Antibody (ANA) Profile. She had been experiencing certain symptoms since May 2015, but they did not seem very troublesome then.

The complaints started with pain in the right knee joint since May 2015. It was sometimes in the right knee and sometimes in the left. Later in December that year, she started getting swelling in her fingers. But since the last 10-15 days, she was experiencing severe knee joint pain and also pain in the joints of her fingers. She also had morning stiffness lasting for about half an hour. Her pain used to get aggravated on walking and also when she used to get up after sitting for long.

About her condition, she said, "I have started feeling very lazy and weak. I always feel like lying down. This physical weakness is overpowering.

Since a few days, even the slightest physical exertion makes me weary. I feel no one should ask me to do any work." Due to the pain she had disturbed sleep. The part on which she lied down had more pain.

On further questioning about any changes that occurred during this time span, she narrated that in January 2015, while teaching in the classroom she had asked a peon to clean the classroom, but he did not listen to her and in turn back answered. She shouted at the peon, and while all this was going on, the principal of the school was passing by their classroom. She enquired what the matter was, and she shouted at her instead of shouting at the peon. From that time, the principal had started targeting her. Furthermore, she also told an instance where once when she was just sitting with her colleague in the staff room, the attendance register was already kept outside before the principal came in. Neither she nor her friend had removed it from the cupboard. Yet the principal started yelling at her asking why she even touched the register in her absence. She also started abusing her in front of all the teachers present in the staff room. To this, she could not do anything. She just started crying.

She further confessed that it was very insulting. She had to listen to unnecessary things for a mistake which she did not even commit. The principal further continued to torture her by changing her shift timings, giving extra work, etc.

The patient admitted that she used to feel angry on seeing her. She was also scared to go to the school for a few days, as she had lost all the respect she once had. She said this incident would always haunt her memory. "Now also if that incident crosses my mind, I feel like crying." She did not like interacting with the principal but was bound to do so. She said those days were very tormenting because no one used to talk to her. So that time she used to feel very isolated and lonely. She could never back-answer her nor did she refrain from doing any extra work given to her. She also went to the school every day even though she was not keeping well.

Now she said, "I have lost interest in work. The same incident keeps on running in my mind. I also avoid talking to anyone. I also used to get angry over my husband and hit my child. Initially, I also worked on holidays when nobody else came to work. I feel even after putting in so many efforts, the principal doesn't understand. She never values my work, never appreciates my efforts."

About her nature, she told us, "I am a person who will get scared if someone shouts at me. I start crying very easily since childhood. I am fearful as a person, and I can't stay alone since childhood nor can I go in the dark. Also I am very fearful before exams. Even if I have to visit any new place, I become scared, and I feel suffocated." She told us that once her brother had scared her in the dark. Following that incident, she fell ill and had to be taken to the hospital.

The patient said, "I am very sensitive. I can't see blood, organs, surgery, horror movies, etc. I did not even go to visit my uncle in the hospital, while he was suffering from pancreatitis. Even on hearing about someone committing suicide, I get afraid. I am very afraid on hearing about kidney diseases because there was a colleague who was going through dialysis. So after hearing about her I also became fearful. I always used to think that I might also contract some kidney disease. I feel because of my disease I will have to remain dependent on other people. And moreover because of these immunosuppressants, I will become more ill. I am also worried about how things will turn out in the future. What will happen to my husband and my kids?"

"Since childhood, I was known as a fearful person. I was also stubborn but only with my parents, not in front of anyone else. For example, I wanted new shoes, but my parents were not agreeing to it, so I bit them. If I wanted some new dress, I wanted it. If not fulfilled, I would start crying. I never got into fights with people. Saying no has been a task for me ever since. I feel the opposite person will be hurt if I say no to them."

During exam time, she said, "I become very restless, and I don't eat or drink anything during that time. I become very scared, and I feel I won't be able to recall anything. But once I see the question paper, I become normal. Even if someone asks for something, I give it away easily. For example, a friend asked for some gold, so I gave it. Even as a kid in school, if someone could not afford to pay their fees, I used to pay for them. I feel sympathetic very easily and give away money even to beggars. I like sleeping a lot. I feel no one should ask me to do any work."

"I had a history of being dominated. It makes me feel very insulted if someone talks to me in a louder tone. My hands and feet start trembling. I got married in 2005. If any of my in-laws said anything, I used to start crying. Even if I used to clean something, my mother-in-law used to come and clean it all over again. That used to make me very angry."

"I am also very concerned about my parents. If they have any tension, I also become stressed. Even when they have any health issues I get concerned and ask them to take proper rest and diet."

"Nowadays, I have started becoming angry. But I express it on my husband and children."

HISTORY FROM HUSBAND:

"She is a helpful person, but is very irritable. Even if she gets angry, it is only expressed in the house, nowhere else."

PHYSICAL GENERALS:

> Appetite: Normal
> Thirst: Thirstless
> Perspiration: Scanty
> Sun: Could not tolerate
> Noise: Did not like. Made her angry
> Tight clothing: Not comfortable
> Sleep: Normal
> Dreams: Not significant
> Thermals: Hot patient

■ SUMMARY OF THE CASE

On tracing the journey of the disease, we could understand that the patient suffered from repeated acute ailments including Tuberculosis while she was 15 years of age. This initiated the process of autoimmunity as a consequence of Mycobacterium induced inappropriate host response to the self-antigen. Thus, the chronicity was reflected in the form of a positive Antinuclear Antibody (ANA) profile at the age of 17 years. It was only after an acute infection of Dengue at the age of 25 years, that the disease flared up in the form of Raynaud's phenomenon, subsequently diagnosed as Systemic Lupus Erythematosus.

Clinical surveillance also suggests that a wide majority of patients suffering from Tuberculosis later contract Wegener's Granulomatosis and Systemic Lupus Erythematosus.

Thus, we can classify this as a miasmatic disease of non-venereal origin, i.e., Psora (For details of the Journey of Disease refer to Chart no. 18). Hence, the affirmations by Dr. Hahnemann in *The Chronic Diseases* still holds true: "Diseases arising from Psora tend to change forms and may reappear with a different name and after a few years with a different set of symptoms."

On analysing the patient as a person, we could cognise that her childhood milieu was one of domination where she was so sensitive that she took every reprimand as an insult and expressed herself only by weeping.

Her disposition also evinced a fearful side, which was seen before exams, visiting a new place, on seeing blood, etc. She was also a kind-hearted person, where she would comply if asked for anything.

Being sensitive as a person, the incident where her principal scolded her without being at fault added fuel to the fire by triggering her core sensitivity of being 'mortified,' which made her symptoms worse. This in turn evoked immense anger in her towards her principal, which was unexpressed at the moment due to lack of courage but was later vented on her husband and children.

This occurrence sensitised her to an extent that even the thought of it made her weep and left an enduring impact where she was even scared of going to school, as she felt she had lost all her respect. Moreover, she felt she was unduly assigned work, which she could not even deny and felt harassed. Over the time, she became sad and started developing an aversion to her work, which she once did very enthusiastically.

Also, one of the regards of the case was her fear and anxiety for her loved ones. The enormity of fear was so much that she would never pay a visit to her relatives admitted in hospital.

▌▌ Rubrics considered were:

> Mind; FEAR dark
> Mind; FEAR alone, of being
> Mind; AILMENTS from mortification, humiliation, chagrin
> Mind; FEAR ghosts, of
> Mind; HORRIBLE things, sad stories affect her profoundly

After contemplating and repertorising the case, remedies which came close were Lycopodium Clavatum, Calcarea Sulphurica, Natrum Muriaticum and Pulsatilla Nigricans.

Natrum Muriaticum, which is in close proximity to the case, was ruled out, as the conflict here was not of relations but of mortification by an authority. The disconcert of Natrum Muriaticum is expecting too much from their close relations, which ultimately leads to disappointment if not adequately met. The plight of Natrum Muraticum is of grief following the departure of "kith and kin" from their life. However, if someone abandons them that very thought clings to their mind but only occasionally awakens the memories of the past. They develop a strong aversion to them, which eventually leads to hatred. One of the significant aggravating modality that we clinically encounter is of consolation aggravation, which arises from a constant feeling of being pitied.

Here, Lycopodium was prescribed because of its sensitivity of being mortified by dominion. There is a constant fear of being mortified which is rooted since childhood due to an upbringing full of domination. The repercussion of this is becoming over-strung at trifles, and they assume that any new task is not their cup of tea, where their core feeling is "Am I capable of doing it?" Although when impelled, they do it with ease. This behaviour runs through the remedy, as they are very low on confidence, which in the long run gives rise to feelings of sadness and melancholy.

Another aspect is their timid behaviour where they fear meeting new acquaintances, and contradictorily, they also fear being alone. Expressing anger only on closed ones also displays a part of their timidity. However, in the compensated state, some Lycopodium patients also appear to be dictatorial and a critic of people around.

Although intellectually very keen, their anxious nature makes them hurried in their daily chores, and they also make mistakes in speaking and writing.

Their demeanour appears to be stern, but they are in fact very tender-hearted on the inside. This pictures itself when they weep on being thanked or give away easily on being flattered.

Although the component of fear prevailed all through the case, the profundity laid in the patient's core sensitivity of being mortified, which swayed our path towards the similimum.

▌▐ REMEDY PRESCRIBED:

➤ Lycopodium Clavatum 200, 1 powder on 17/05/2016

▌▐ Patient came to us with the following reports: 06/05/2016

➤ Hb: 10.2 gm/dl
➤ ESR: 65 mm at the end of 1 hour
➤ C-Reactive Protein: Reactive

> ANA Profile:
  - Result - Positive
  - Pattern - Speckled
  - Grade - +++
  - Estimated Titre - 1:1000

▌█ FOLLOW-UPS:

31/05/2016

> Bilateral knee pain was better; there was swelling on and off.

> Due to the summer heat, was not able to sleep.

> Headache since 2 days.

> Overall pain was better now.

▌█ PRESCRIPTION: Placebo.

12/07/2016

> Death of a cousin, due to which she had suicidal thoughts. Sleep was disturbed.

> Morning stiffness was better. Knee pain was better. Had pain on and off.

> Frequency of headache had increased.

> On examination: Peripheral cyanosis was present.

▌█ PRESCRIPTION: Placebo.

30/07/2016

> Sleep disturbance still persisted.

> Pain in upper extremities was better. Morning stiffness also better than before.

> Knee pain had started again, after the death of the cousin.

> Mentally, she did not feel like doing any work.

Reports done during the course of treatment 28/07/2016:

- Hb: 11.9 gm/dl
- ESR: 41 mm at the end of 1 hour
- C-Reactive Protein: Non-Reactive
- ANA Profile:
  - Result - Positive
  - Pattern - Speckled
  - Grade - ++
  - Estimated Titre - 1:320

ANA profile – DNA (Double strand antibody) NcX- Negative (69.17 IU/mL)

▌▌ PRESCRIPTION: Placebo

02/09/2016:

- She said she got irritated very easily now. Did not like any noise.
- Knee pain had also increased, but the morning stiffness was better.
- Bluish discoloration on palms due to cold weather.
- Did not like to go out in public. Also, she still had suicidal thoughts.

▌▌ PRESCRIPTION: Lycopodium Clavatum 200, 1 powder was given

05/10/2016:

- Morning stiffness was much better. The knee pain had also reduced.
- Feeling weak; had one episode of headache for which she took a painkiller.
- Mentally, still felt like not meeting people and stayed back home all the time.
- Peripheral Cyanosis better.

▌▌ PRESCRIPTION: Lycopodium Clavatum 1M, 1 powder was given

NOTE: As the patient was not showing a desired mental improvement, the potency of the remedy was increased.

After that, she continued with the follow-up. She improved mentally. Her pain and morning stiffness were also much better now. There was reduction in the peripheral cyanosis as well.

SCHEMATIC REPRESENTATIONS: JOURNEY OF CHRONIC DISEASES

CHART NO. 1

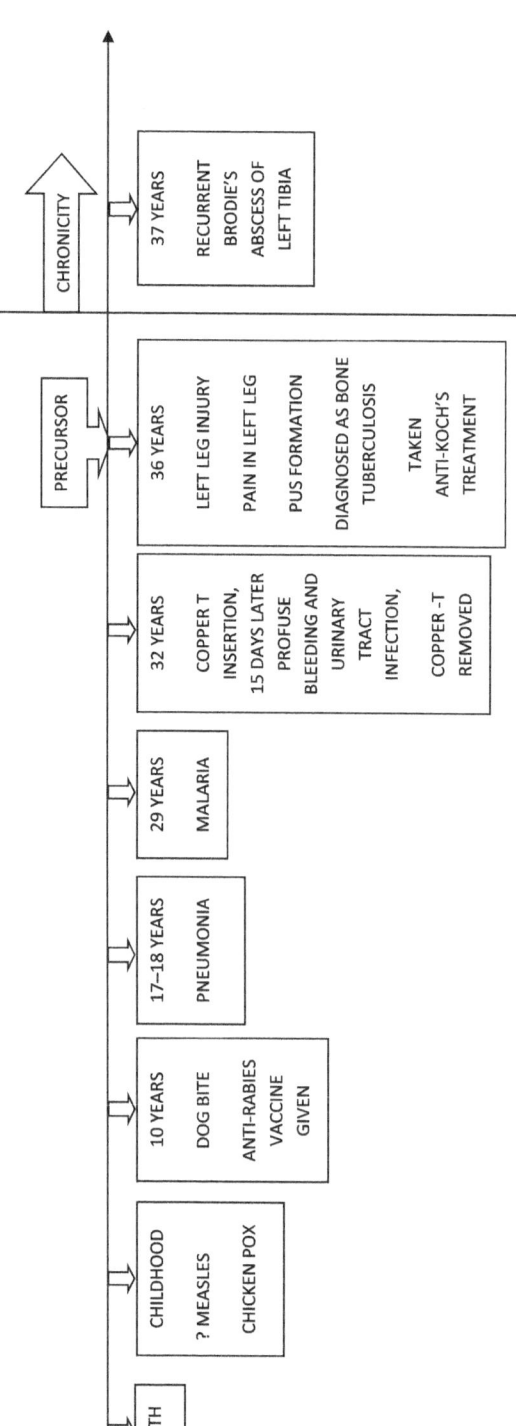

| BIRTH | CHILDHOOD

? MEASLES

CHICKEN POX | 10 YEARS

DOG BITE

ANTI-RABIES VACCINE GIVEN | 17–18 YEARS

PNEUMONIA | 29 YEARS

MALARIA | 32 YEARS

COPPER T INSERTION,

15 DAYS LATER PROFUSE BLEEDING AND URINARY TRACT INFECTION,

COPPER -T REMOVED | 36 YEARS

LEFT LEG INJURY

PAIN IN LEFT LEG

PUS FORMATION

DIAGNOSED AS BONE TUBERCULOSIS

TAKEN ANTI-KOCH'S TREATMENT | 37 YEARS

RECURRENT BRODIE'S ABSCESS OF LEFT TIBIA |

PRECURSOR

CHRONICITY

- CHRONIC MIASMATIC DISEASE - NON VENEREAL IN ORIGIN.
- Here, the precursor is tuberculosis, as till then the patient only had infections at certain phases of life and suffered from no chronic diseases.
- Also, the profuse bleeding after Copper T insertion was just an indisposition which stopped after removal of the Copper T.

CHART NO. 2

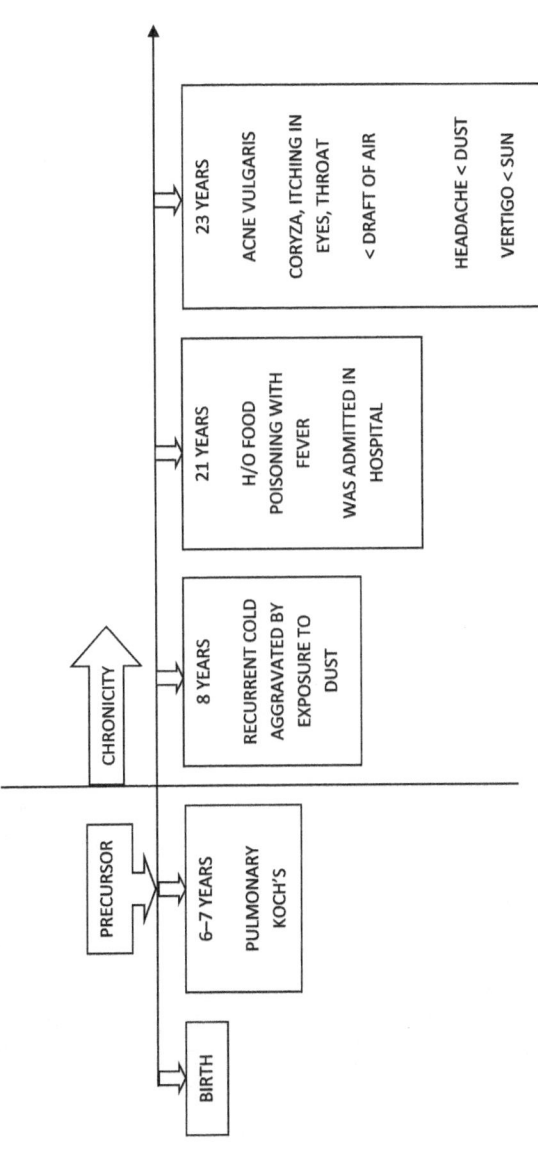

- **CHRONIC MIASMATIC DISEASE – NON VENEREAL IN ORIGIN.**
- Precursor here is Pulmonary Tuberculosis. Following this infection, she suffered from recurrent cold and cough (allergy), which in itself is a form of chronicity.

CHART NO. 3

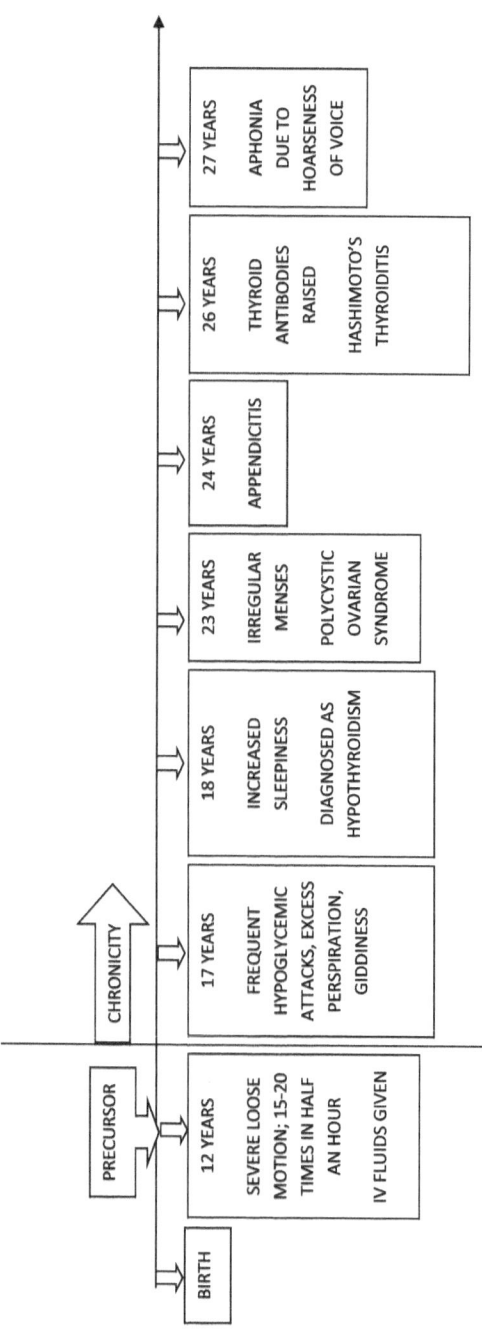

- CHRONIC MIASMATIC DISEASE – NON VENEREAL IN ORIGIN.
- In the above case, severe loose motion (Gastroenteritis) led to disturbance in the body, which later manifested in the form of chronicity by affecting the thyroid gland, irregular menstrual cycle, etc.
  - This case is a classical example of the declaration by Dr Hahnemann: "Diseases arising from Psora tend to change forms and may appear with a different name and after few years with a different set of symptoms."

CHART NO. 4

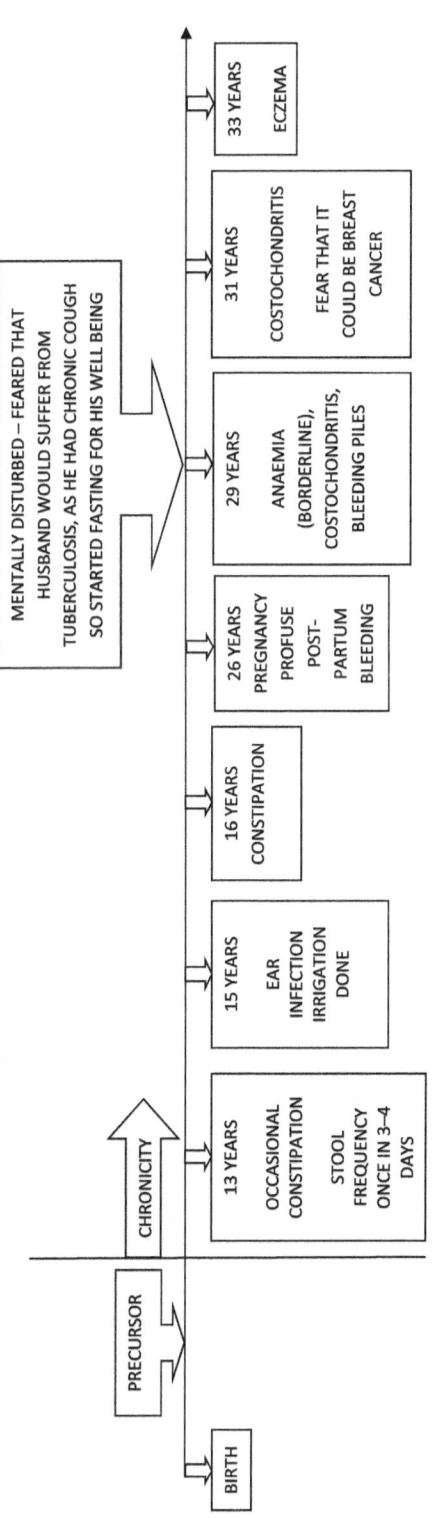

PRECURSOR

CHRONICITY

BIRTH

13 YEARS

OCCASIONAL CONSTIPATION

STOOL FREQUENCY ONCE IN 3–4 DAYS

15 YEARS

EAR INFECTION IRRIGATION DONE

16 YEARS CONSTIPATION

26 YEARS

PREGNANCY PROFUSE POST-PARTUM BLEEDING

29 YEARS

ANAEMIA (BORDERLINE), COSTOCHONDRITIS, BLEEDING PILES

31 YEARS

COSTOCHONDRITIS

FEAR THAT IT COULD BE BREAST CANCER

33 YEARS

ECZEMA

MENTALLY DISTURBED – FEARED THAT HUSBAND WOULD SUFFER FROM TUBERCULOSIS, AS HE HAD CHRONIC COUGH SO STARTED FASTING FOR HIS WELL BEING

• PRECURSOR NOT TRACED.

CHART NO. 5

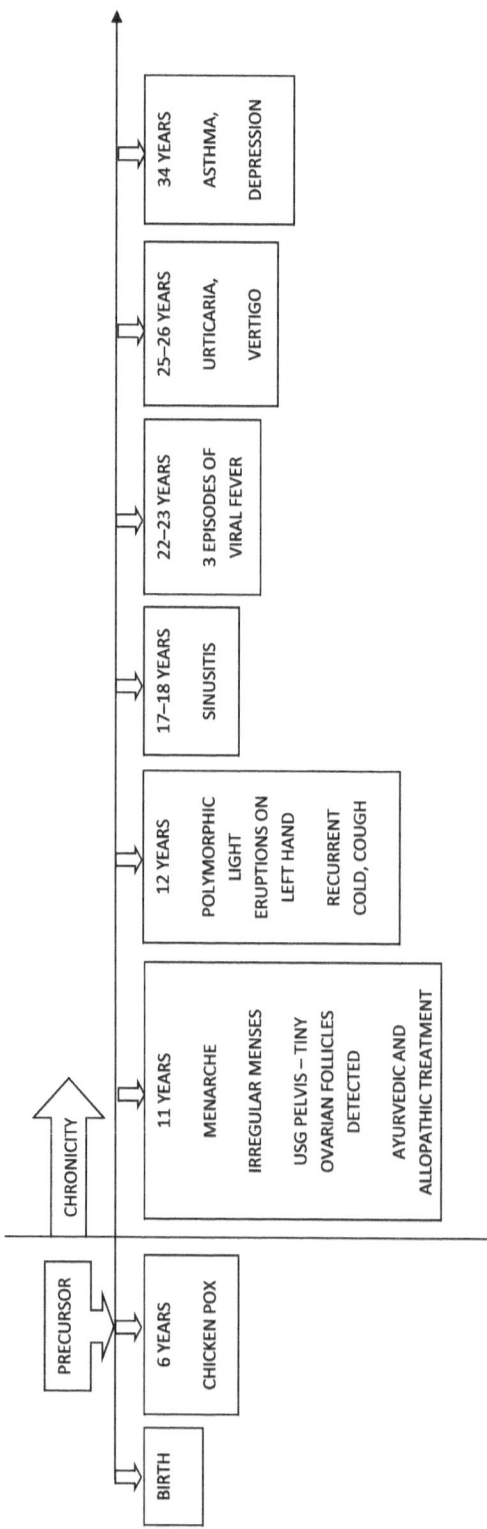

- **CHRONIC MIASMATIC DISEASE – NON VENEREAL IN ORIGIN.**
- Precursor for chronicity is Chicken Pox, which led to irregular menses and Polymorphic Light Eruptions, which was later followed by Urticaria, Asthma and Depression.

BIRTH

PRECURSOR

6 YEARS

CHICKEN POX

CHRONICITY

11 YEARS

MENARCHE

IRREGULAR MENSES

USG PELVIS – TINY OVARIAN FOLLICLES DETECTED

AYURVEDIC AND ALLOPATHIC TREATMENT

12 YEARS

POLYMORPHIC LIGHT ERUPTIONS ON LEFT HAND

RECURRENT COLD, COUGH

17–18 YEARS

SINUSITIS

22–23 YEARS

3 EPISODES OF VIRAL FEVER

25–26 YEARS

URTICARIA, VERTIGO

34 YEARS

ASTHMA, DEPRESSION

CHART NO. 6

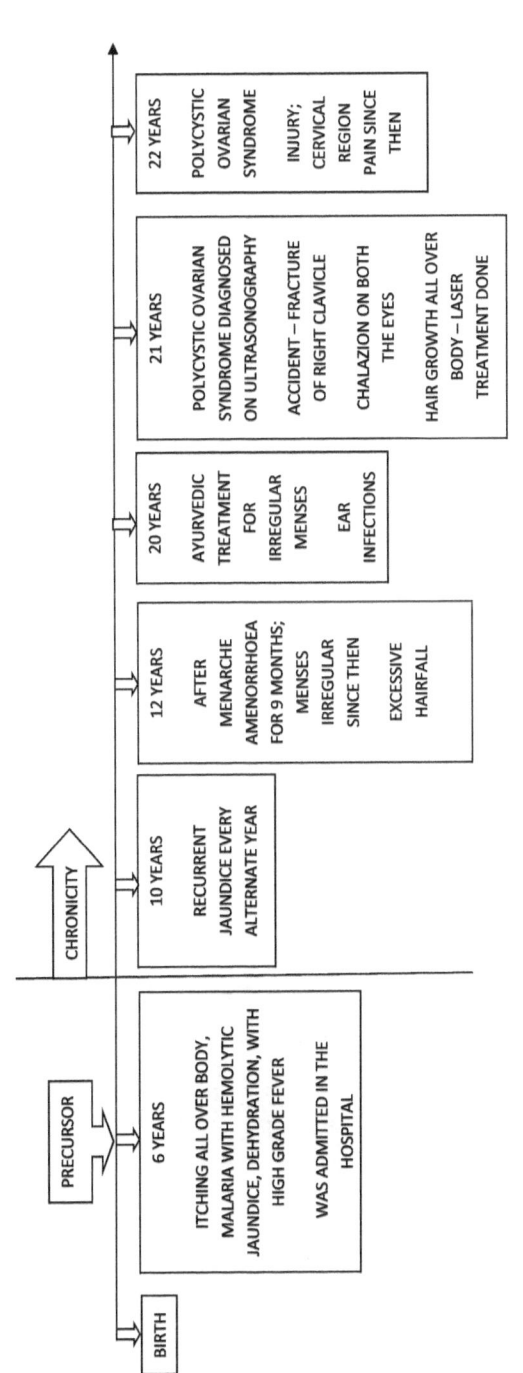

BIRTH	PRECURSOR		CHRONICITY				
	6 YEARS	10 YEARS	12 YEARS	20 YEARS	21 YEARS	22 YEARS
	ITCHING ALL OVER BODY, MALARIA WITH HEMOLYTIC JAUNDICE, DEHYDRATION, WITH HIGH GRADE FEVER	RECURRENT JAUNDICE EVERY ALTERNATE YEAR	AFTER MENARCHE AMENORRHOEA FOR 9 MONTHS; MENSES IRREGULAR SINCE THEN	AYURVEDIC TREATMENT FOR IRREGULAR MENSES	POLYCYSTIC OVARIAN SYNDROME DIAGNOSED ON ULTRASONOGRAPHY	POLYCYSTIC OVARIAN SYNDROME
	WAS ADMITTED IN THE HOSPITAL		EXCESSIVE HAIRFALL	EAR INFECTIONS	ACCIDENT – FRACTURE OF RIGHT CLAVICLE	INJURY; CERVICAL REGION PAIN SINCE THEN
					CHALAZION ON BOTH THE EYES	
					HAIR GROWTH ALL OVER BODY – LASER TREATMENT DONE	

- CHRONIC MIASMATIC DISEASE – NON VENEREAL IN ORIGIN.
- EXPLANATION GIVEN IN CASE NO. 3.

CHART NO. 7

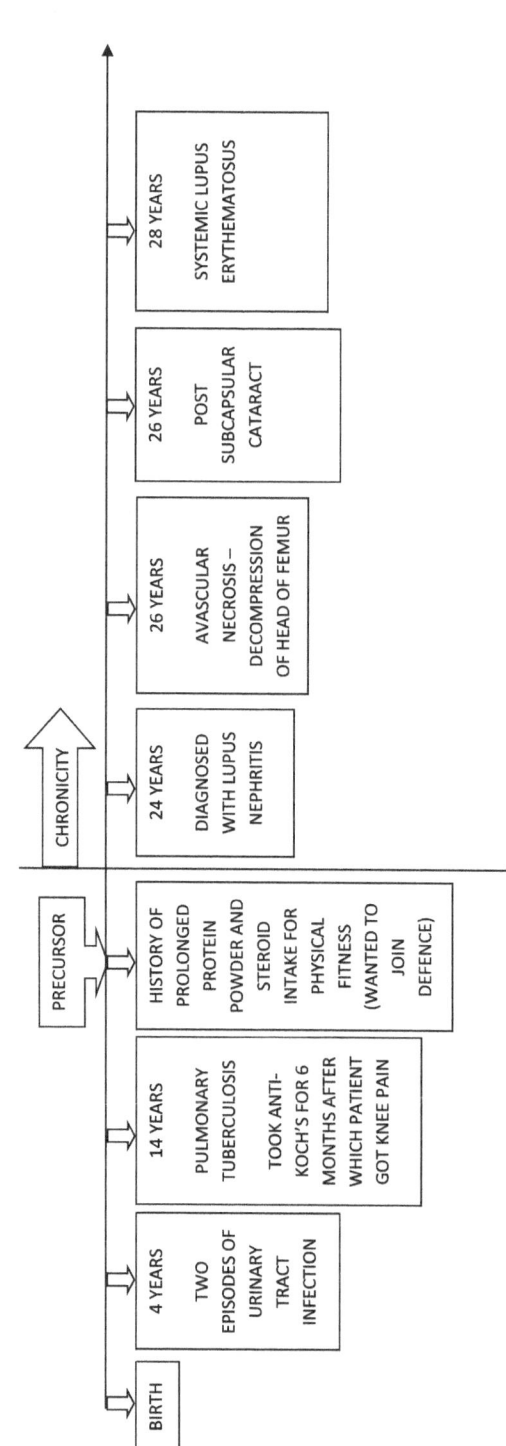

BIRTH

4 YEARS — TWO EPISODES OF URINARY TRACT INFECTION

14 YEARS — PULMONARY TUBERCULOSIS — TOOK ANTI-KOCH'S FOR 6 MONTHS AFTER WHICH PATIENT GOT KNEE PAIN

PRECURSOR

HISTORY OF PROLONGED PROTEIN POWDER AND STEROID INTAKE FOR PHYSICAL FITNESS (WANTED TO JOIN DEFENCE)

CHRONICITY

24 YEARS — DIAGNOSED WITH LUPUS NEPHRITIS

26 YEARS — AVASCULAR NECROSIS – DECOMPRESSION OF HEAD OF FEMUR

26 YEARS — POST SUBCAPSULAR CATARACT

28 YEARS — SYSTEMIC LUPUS ERYTHEMATOSUS

- NON MIASMATIC – ARTIFICIAL CHRONIC DISEASE.
- The prolonged intake of artificial protein and steroid triggered the process of autoimmunity leading to Lupus Nephritis, the after-effects of which manifested as Avascular Necrosis, Subcapsular Cataract and Systemic Lupus Erythematosus.

CHART NO. 8

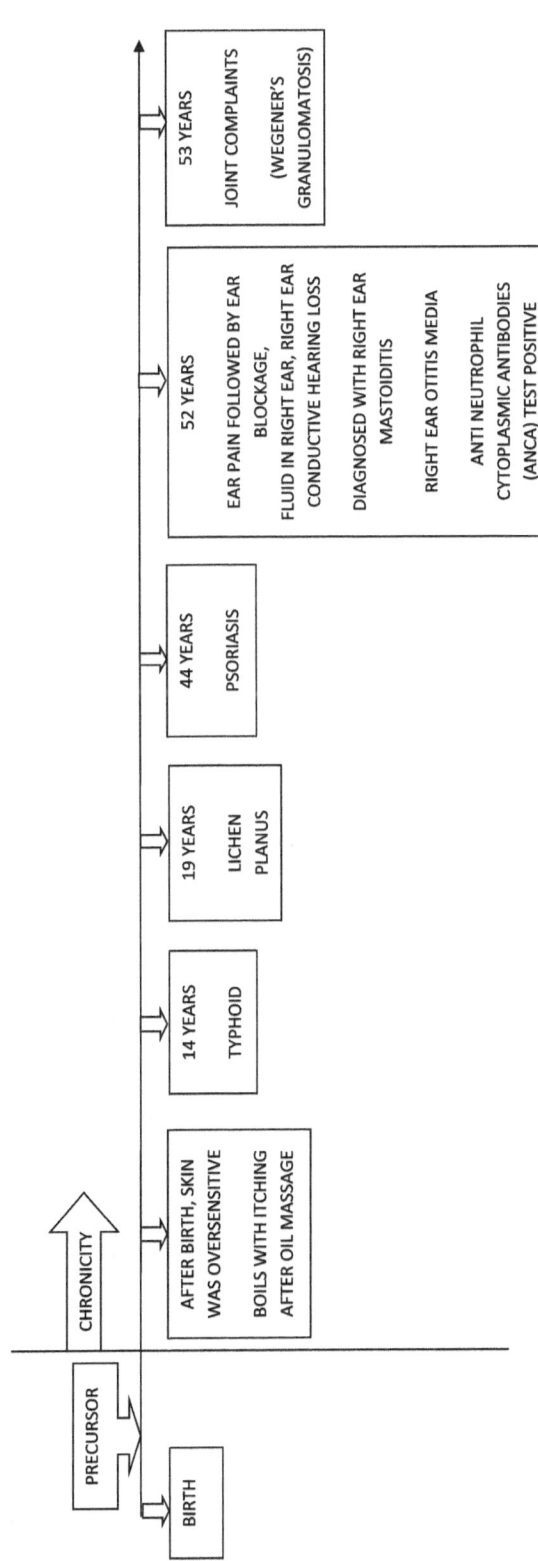

PRECURSOR → **BIRTH**

CHRONICITY

AFTER BIRTH, SKIN WAS OVERSENSITIVE

BOILS WITH ITCHING AFTER OIL MASSAGE

14 YEARS

TYPHOID

19 YEARS

LICHEN PLANUS

44 YEARS

PSORIASIS

52 YEARS

EAR PAIN FOLLOWED BY EAR BLOCKAGE,

FLUID IN RIGHT EAR, RIGHT EAR CONDUCTIVE HEARING LOSS

DIAGNOSED WITH RIGHT EAR MASTOIDITIS

RIGHT EAR OTITIS MEDIA

ANTI NEUTROPHIL CYTOPLASMIC ANTIBODIES (ANCA) TEST POSITIVE

53 YEARS

JOINT COMPLAINTS

(WEGENER'S GRANULOMATOSIS)

- PRECURSOR NOT TRACED.

- In a few months after birth, over sensitiveness of skin was observed, which indicated allergic reaction, which itself is a form of chronicity. So, there has to be a precursor before that, which is likely to be vaccination, which has high tendency to create skin allergy.

CHART NO. 9

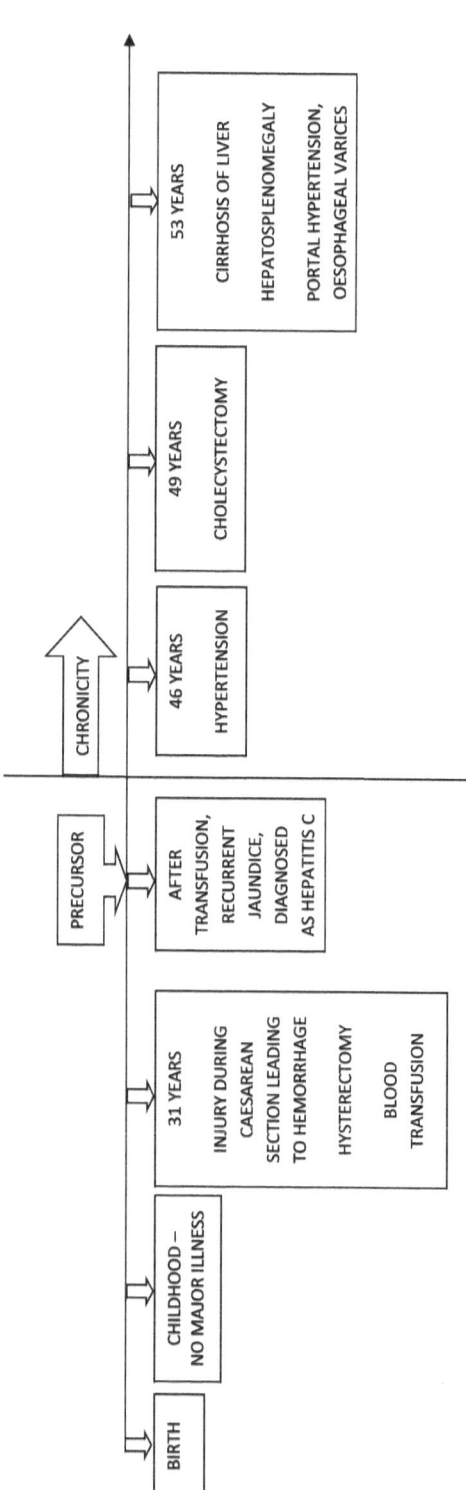

- CHRONIC MIASMATIC DISEASE – VENEREAL IN ORIGIN.

- Although the route of transmission of the infection was through blood transfusion (manmade route), Hepatitis C can naturally be transmitted only through venereal source.

- Cirrhosis of Liver is a result of the already contracted venereal infection (Hepatitis C).

- In venereal-originating diseases, the precursor (organism) can always be traced in the body, which is not the scenario in non-venereal originating diseases and is the major differentiating point between them.

The following text appears within the chart:

BIRTH

CHILDHOOD – NO MAJOR ILLNESS

31 YEARS

INJURY DURING CAESAREAN SECTION LEADING TO HEMORRHAGE

HYSTERECTOMY

BLOOD TRANSFUSION

PRECURSOR

AFTER TRANSFUSION, RECURRENT JAUNDICE, DIAGNOSED AS HEPATITIS C

CHRONICITY

46 YEARS

HYPERTENSION

49 YEARS

CHOLECYSTECTOMY

53 YEARS

CIRRHOSIS OF LIVER

HEPATOSPLENOMEGALY

PORTAL HYPERTENSION, OESOPHAGEAL VARICES

CHART NO. 10

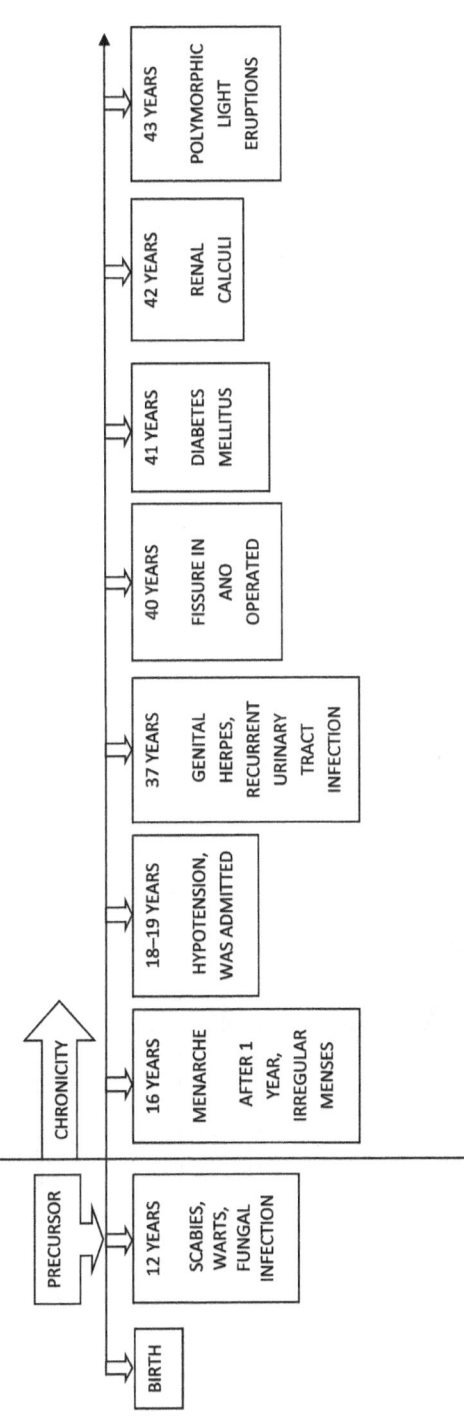

- CHRONIC MIASMATIC DISEASE – NON VENEREAL IN ORIGIN.
- The precursor here was scabies and fungal infection, which initiated the process of chronicity in the form of Menstrual Irregularities, Diabetes Mellitus, Renal Calculi and Polymorphic Light Eruptions.
  - Here, although the patient suffered from Genital Herpes, it was only an opportunistic infection and not the precursor, as the chronicity had already set in after scabies and fungal infection.

CHART NO. 11

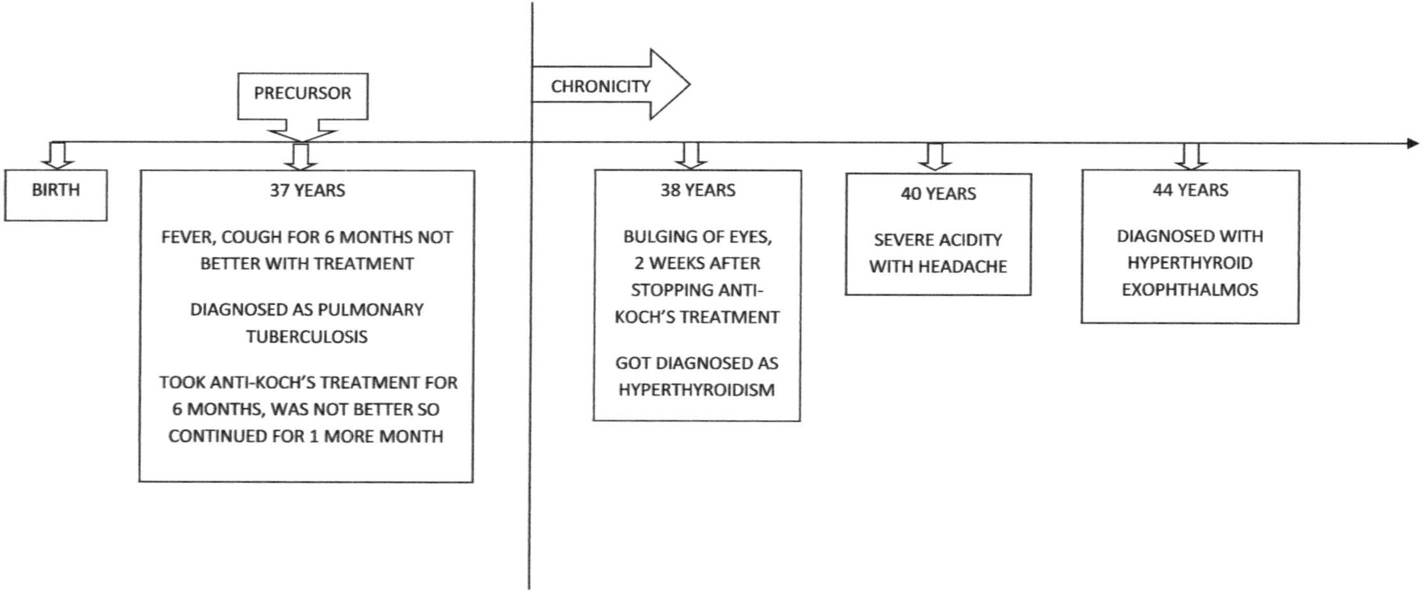

BIRTH

PRECURSOR

CHRONICITY

37 YEARS

FEVER, COUGH FOR 6 MONTHS NOT BETTER WITH TREATMENT

DIAGNOSED AS PULMONARY TUBERCULOSIS

TOOK ANTI-KOCH'S TREATMENT FOR 6 MONTHS, WAS NOT BETTER SO CONTINUED FOR 1 MORE MONTH

38 YEARS

BULGING OF EYES, 2 WEEKS AFTER STOPPING ANTI-KOCH'S TREATMENT

GOT DIAGNOSED AS HYPERTHYROIDISM

40 YEARS

SEVERE ACIDITY WITH HEADACHE

44 YEARS

DIAGNOSED WITH HYPERTHYROID EXOPHTHALMOS

- MIASMATIC CHRONIC DISEASE – NON VENEREAL IN ORIGIN.
- The primary infection of Pulmonary Koch's has led to autoimmune process giving rise to Hyperthyroidism.
- EXPLANATION GIVEN IN CASE NO. 2.

CHART NO. 12

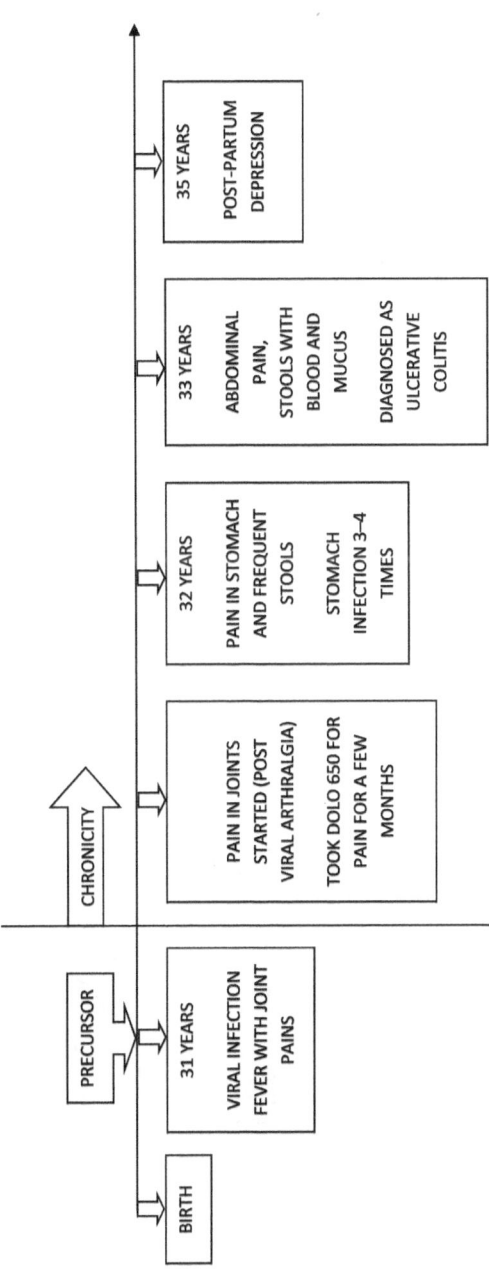

- CHRONIC MIASMATIC DISEASE – NON VENEREAL IN ORIGIN.
- The precursor is viral fever, which initiated the joint pains. The pain killers taken for joint pains made the gastrointestinal lining sensitive, which acted as an exciting cause for stomach infections and further Ulcerative Colitis.

CHART NO. 13

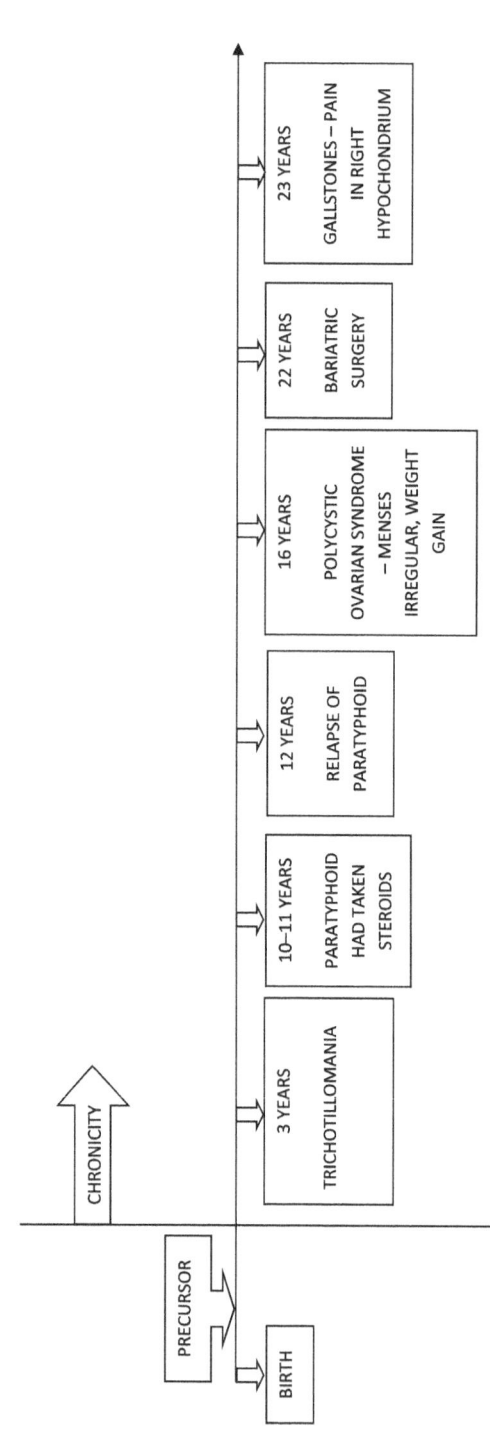

- PRECURSOR NOT TRACED.
- Trichotillomania indicated mental disorder at 3 years of age, which has an unidentified precursor in the background.

CHART NO. 14

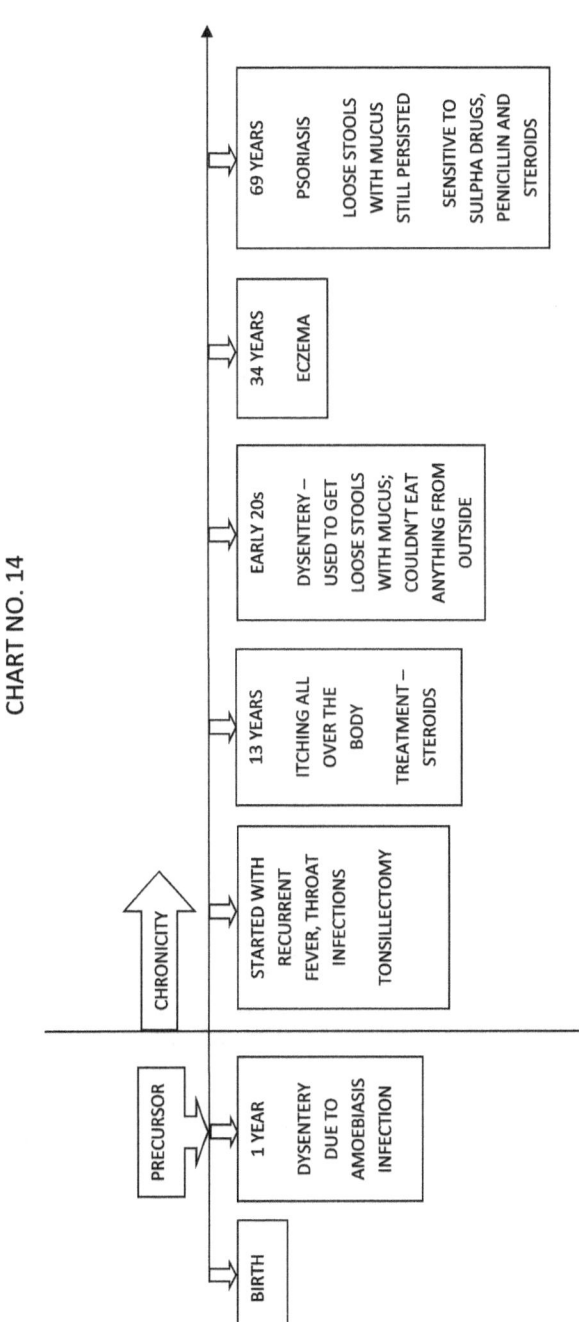

- **CHRONIC MIASMATIC DISEASE – NON VENEREAL IN ORIGIN.**
- The precursor here is Amoebiasis which led to chronic diseases like Psoriasis and loose stools with mucus (?Inflammatory Bowel Disease).

CHART NO. 15

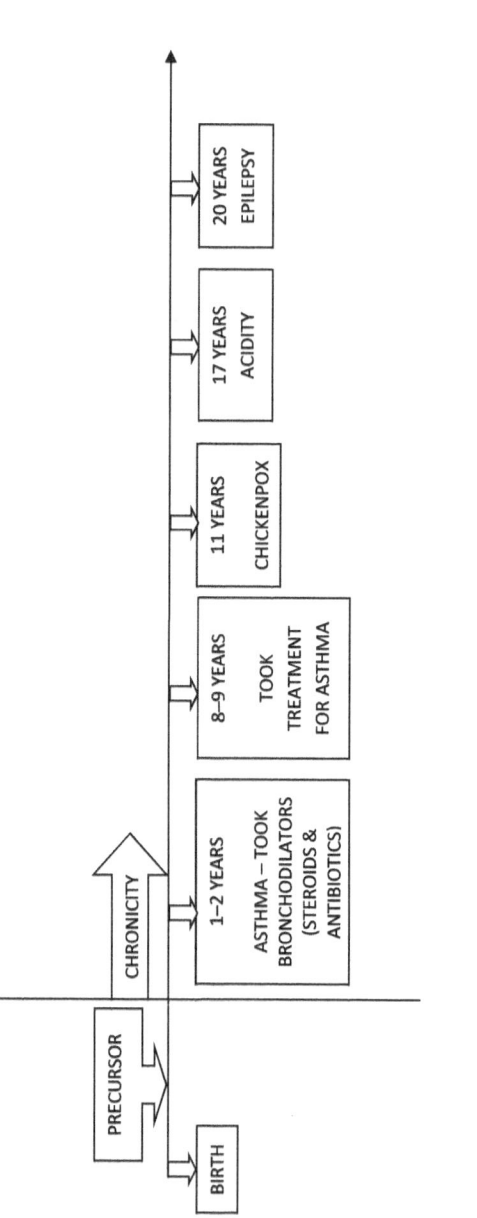

- PRECURSOR NOT TRACED.
- Asthma itself indicates chronicity, which was already present since the age of 1–2 years.

CHART NO. 16

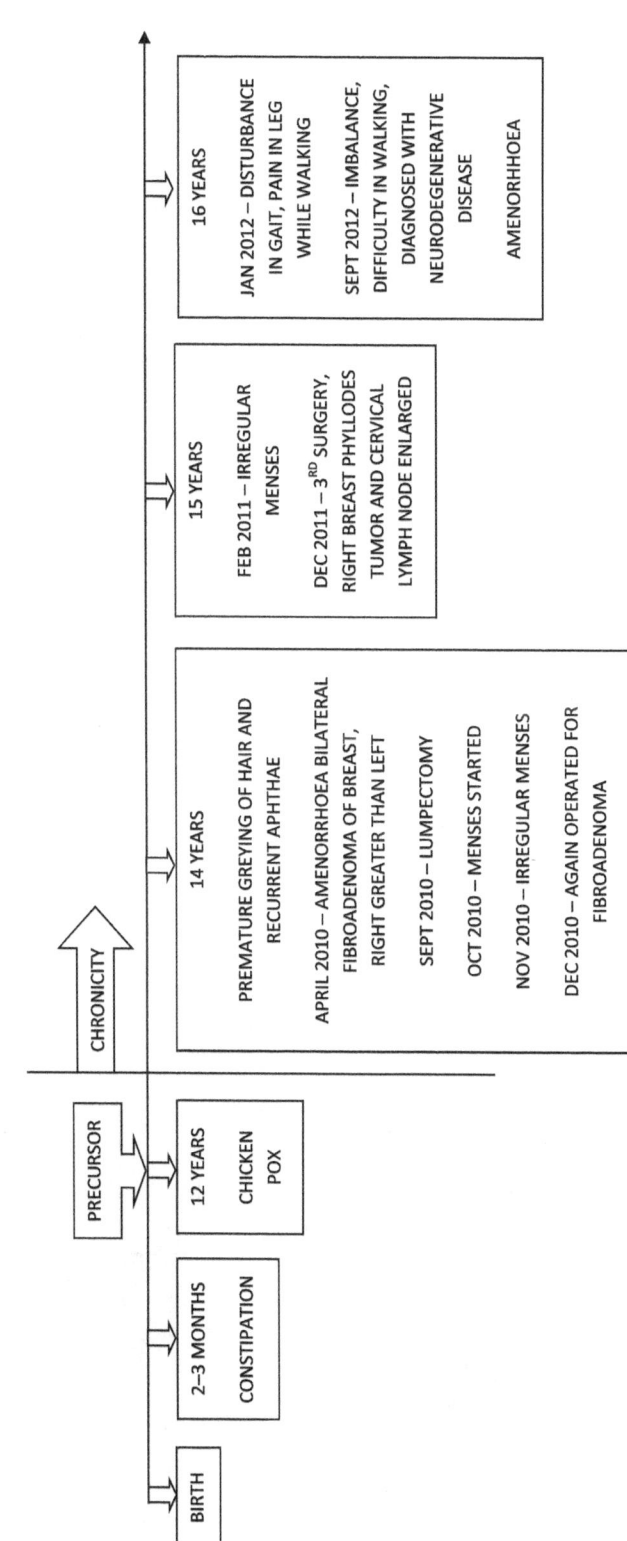

BIRTH

2–3 MONTHS — CONSTIPATION

PRECURSOR

12 YEARS — CHICKEN POX

CHRONICITY

14 YEARS

PREMATURE GREYING OF HAIR AND RECURRENT APHTHAE

APRIL 2010 – AMENORRHOEA BILATERAL FIBROADENOMA OF BREAST, RIGHT GREATER THAN LEFT

SEPT 2010 – LUMPECTOMY

OCT 2010 – MENSES STARTED

NOV 2010 – IRREGULAR MENSES

DEC 2010 – AGAIN OPERATED FOR FIBROADENOMA

15 YEARS

FEB 2011 – IRREGULAR MENSES

DEC 2011 – 3RD SURGERY, RIGHT BREAST PHYLLODES TUMOR AND CERVICAL LYMPH NODE ENLARGED

16 YEARS

JAN 2012 – DISTURBANCE IN GAIT, PAIN IN LEG WHILE WALKING

SEPT 2012 – IMBALANCE, DIFFICULTY IN WALKING, DIAGNOSED WITH NEURODEGENERATIVE DISEASE

AMENORRHOEA

- CHRONIC MIASMATIC DISEASE – NON VENEREAL IN ORIGIN.
- EXPLANATION GIVEN IN CASE NO. 1.

CHART NO. 17

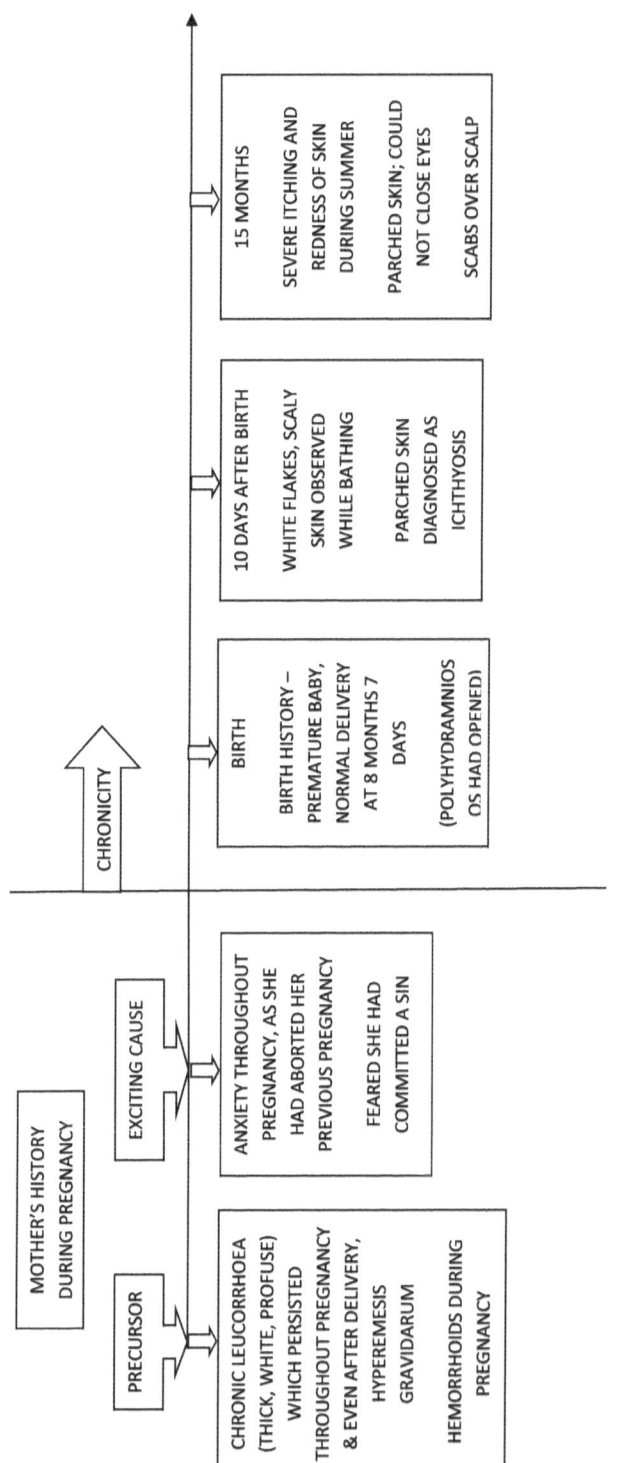

MOTHER'S HISTORY DURING PREGNANCY

PRECURSOR

CHRONIC LEUCORRHOEA (THICK, WHITE, PROFUSE) WHICH PERSISTED THROUGHOUT PREGNANCY & EVEN AFTER DELIVERY, HYPEREMESIS GRAVIDARUM

HEMORRHOIDS DURING PREGNANCY

EXCITING CAUSE

ANXIETY THROUGHOUT PREGNANCY, AS SHE HAD ABORTED HER PREVIOUS PREGNANCY

FEARED SHE HAD COMMITTED A SIN

CHRONICITY

BIRTH

BIRTH HISTORY – PREMATURE BABY, NORMAL DELIVERY AT 8 MONTHS 7 DAYS

(POLYHYDRAMNIOS OS HAD OPENED)

10 DAYS AFTER BIRTH

WHITE FLAKES, SCALY SKIN OBSERVED WHILE BATHING

PARCHED SKIN DIAGNOSED AS ICHTHYOSIS

15 MONTHS

SEVERE ITCHING AND REDNESS OF SKIN DURING SUMMER

PARCHED SKIN; COULD NOT CLOSE EYES

SCABS OVER SCALP

- CHRONIC MIASMATIC DISEASE – VENEREAL IN ORIGIN.
- EXPLANATION GIVEN IN CASE NO. 9.

CHART NO. 18

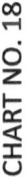

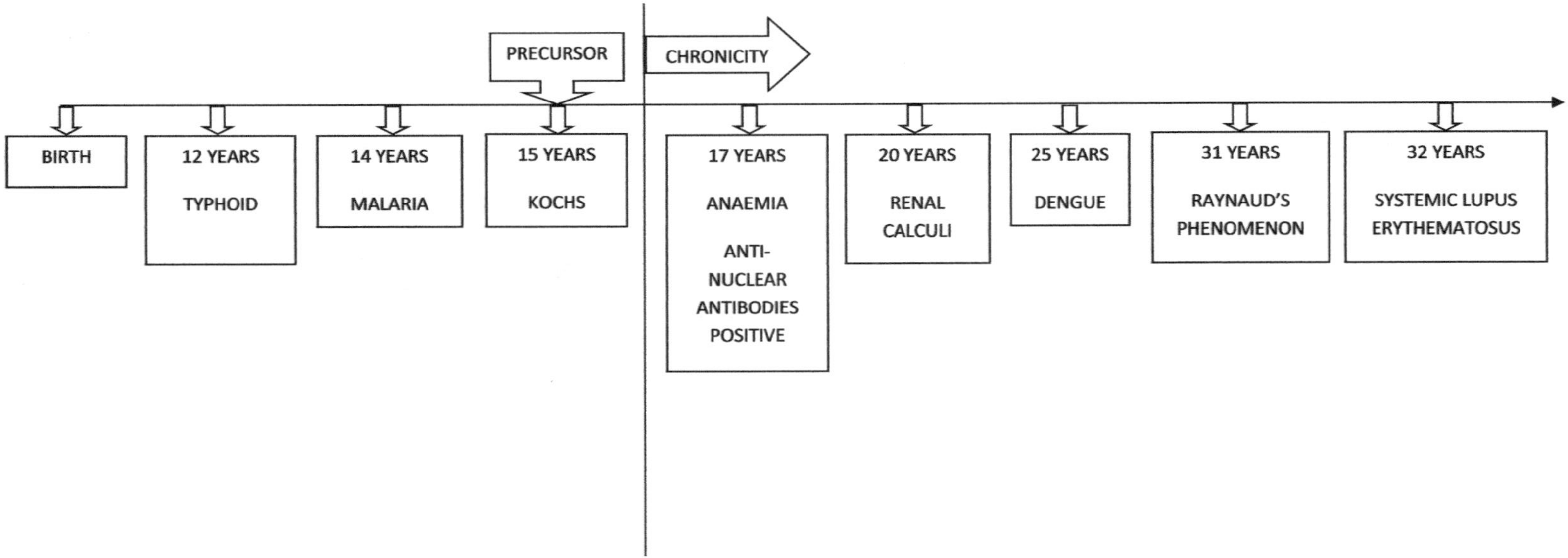

BIRTH	12 YEARS TYPHOID	14 YEARS MALARIA	15 YEARS KOCHS	17 YEARS ANAEMIA ANTI-NUCLEAR ANTIBODIES POSITIVE	20 YEARS RENAL CALCULI	25 YEARS DENGUE	31 YEARS RAYNAUD'S PHENOMENON	32 YEARS SYSTEMIC LUPUS ERYTHEMATOSUS

PRECURSOR

CHRONICITY

- CHRONIC MIASMATIC DISEASE – NON VENEREAL IN ORIGIN.
- EXPLANATION GIVEN IN CASE NO. 10.

CHART NO. 19

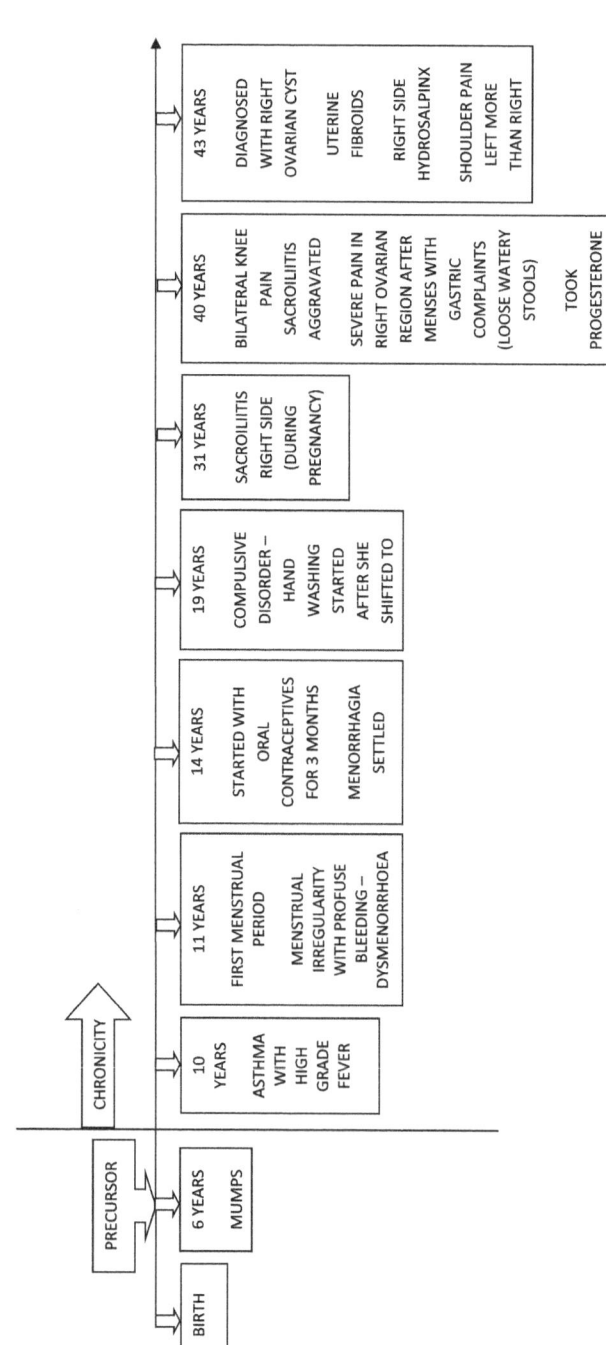

BIRTH	6 YEARS	10 YEARS	11 YEARS	14 YEARS	19 YEARS	31 YEARS	40 YEARS	43 YEARS
	MUMPS	ASTHMA WITH HIGH GRADE FEVER	FIRST MENSTRUAL PERIOD MENSTRUAL IRREGULARITY WITH PROFUSE BLEEDING – DYSMENORRHOEA	STARTED WITH ORAL CONTRACEPTIVES FOR 3 MONTHS MENORRHAGIA SETTLED	COMPULSIVE DISORDER – HAND WASHING STARTED AFTER SHE SHIFTED TO	SACROILIITIS RIGHT SIDE (DURING PREGNANCY)	BILATERAL KNEE PAIN SACROILIITIS AGGRAVATED SEVERE PAIN IN RIGHT OVARIAN REGION AFTER MENSES WITH GASTRIC COMPLAINTS (LOOSE WATERY STOOLS) TOOK PROGESTERONE	DIAGNOSED WITH RIGHT OVARIAN CYST UTERINE FIBROIDS RIGHT SIDE HYDROSALPINX SHOULDER PAIN LEFT MORE THAN RIGHT

PRECURSOR

CHRONICITY

- CHRONIC MIASMATIC DISEASE – NON VENEREAL IN ORIGIN.
- Mumps acted as the precursor, which initiated the process of chronicity. Thus, Dr. Hahnemann has rightly stated Psora as being hydra-headed which tends to exhibit its varied forms along the years.

CHART NO. 20

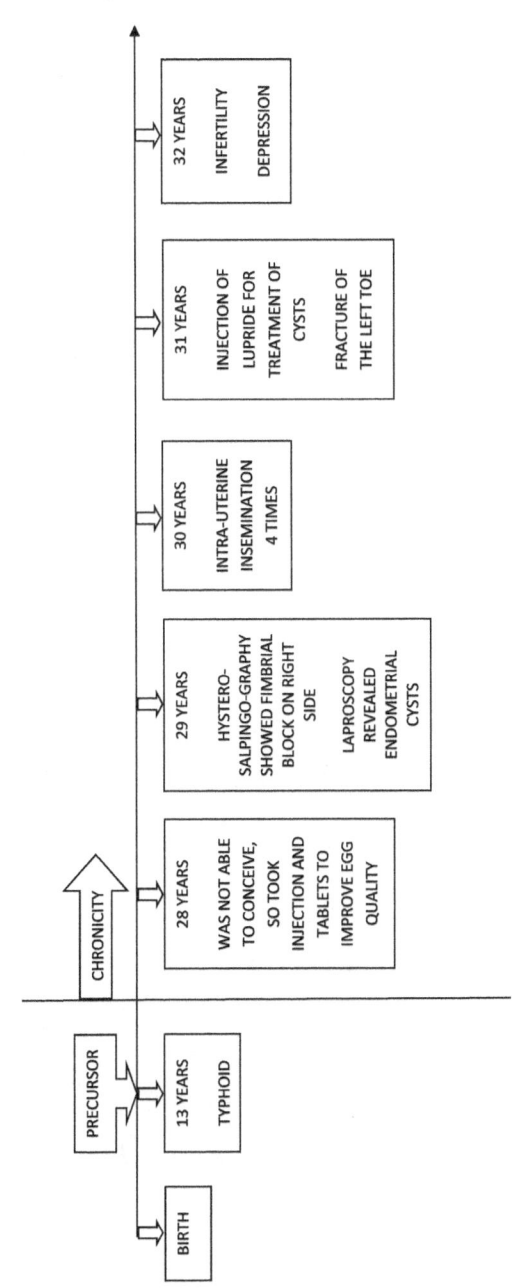

- CHRONIC MIASMATIC DISEASE – NON VENEREAL IN ORIGIN.
- Here the precursor is Typhoid leading to Infertility and Depression.

CHART NO. 21

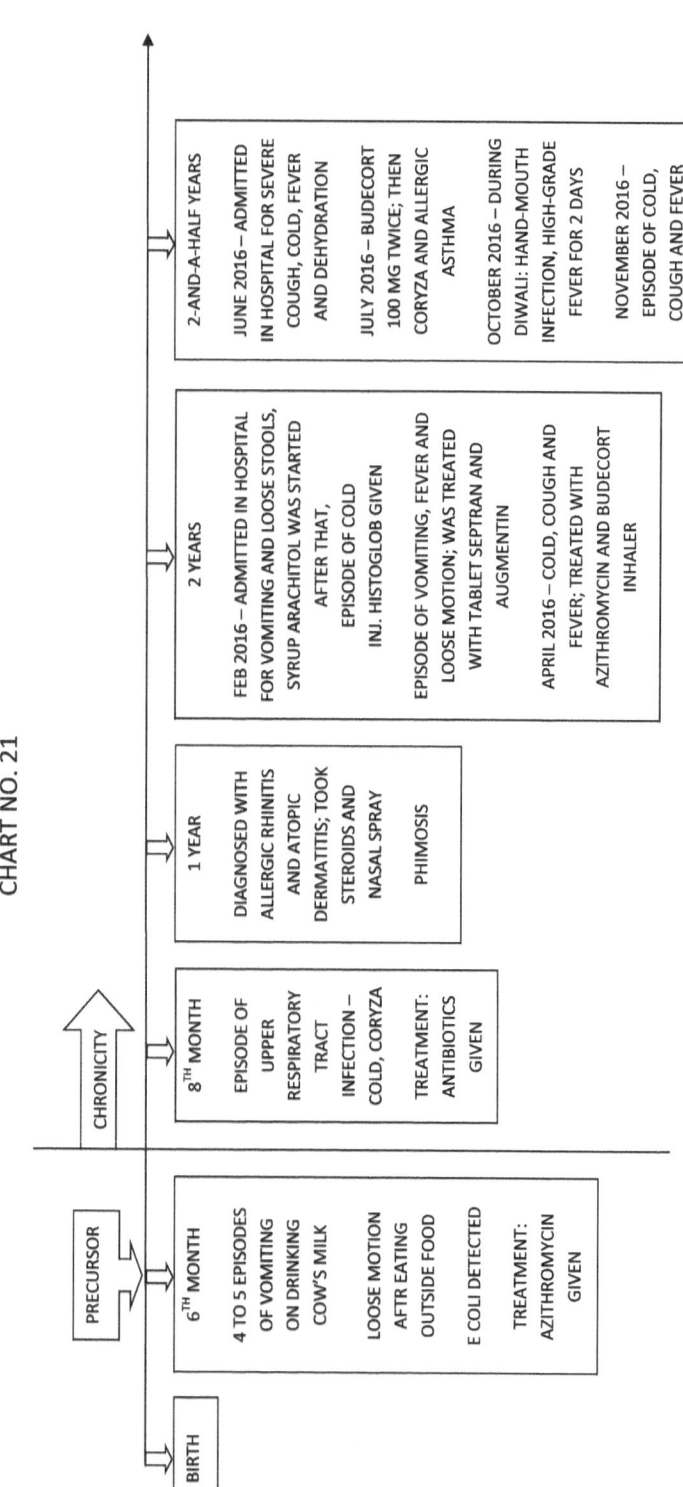

BIRTH

PRECURSOR

CHRONICITY

6TH MONTH

4 TO 5 EPISODES OF VOMITING ON DRINKING COW'S MILK

LOOSE MOTION AFTR EATING OUTSIDE FOOD

E COLI DETECTED

TREATMENT: AZITHROMYCIN GIVEN

8TH MONTH

EPISODE OF UPPER RESPIRATORY TRACT INFECTION – COLD, CORYZA

TREATMENT: ANTIBIOTICS GIVEN

1 YEAR

DIAGNOSED WITH ALLERGIC RHINITIS AND ATOPIC DERMATITIS; TOOK STEROIDS AND NASAL SPRAY

PHIMOSIS

2 YEARS

FEB 2016 – ADMITTED IN HOSPITAL FOR VOMITING AND LOOSE STOOLS, SYRUP ARACHITOL WAS STARTED AFTER THAT, EPISODE OF COLD INJ. HISTOGLOB GIVEN

EPISODE OF VOMITING, FEVER AND LOOSE MOTION; WAS TREATED WITH TABLET SEPTRAN AND AUGMENTIN

APRIL 2016 – COLD, COUGH AND FEVER; TREATED WITH AZITHROMYCIN AND BUDECORT INHALER

2-AND-A-HALF YEARS

JUNE 2016 – ADMITTED IN HOSPITAL FOR SEVERE COUGH, COLD, FEVER AND DEHYDRATION

JULY 2016 – BUDECORT 100 MG TWICE; THEN CORYZA AND ALLERGIC ASTHMA

OCTOBER 2016 – DURING DIWALI: HAND-MOUTH INFECTION, HIGH-GRADE FEVER FOR 2 DAYS

NOVEMBER 2016 – EPISODE OF COLD, COUGH AND FEVER

- CHRONIC MIASMATIC DISEASE – NON VENEREAL IN ORIGIN.
- Here E. Coli, which was introduced in the body through cow's milk, served as a precursor and induced chronicity in the form of recurrent Upper Respiratory Tract Infections and Gastrointestinal Affections in the child.

CHART NO. 22

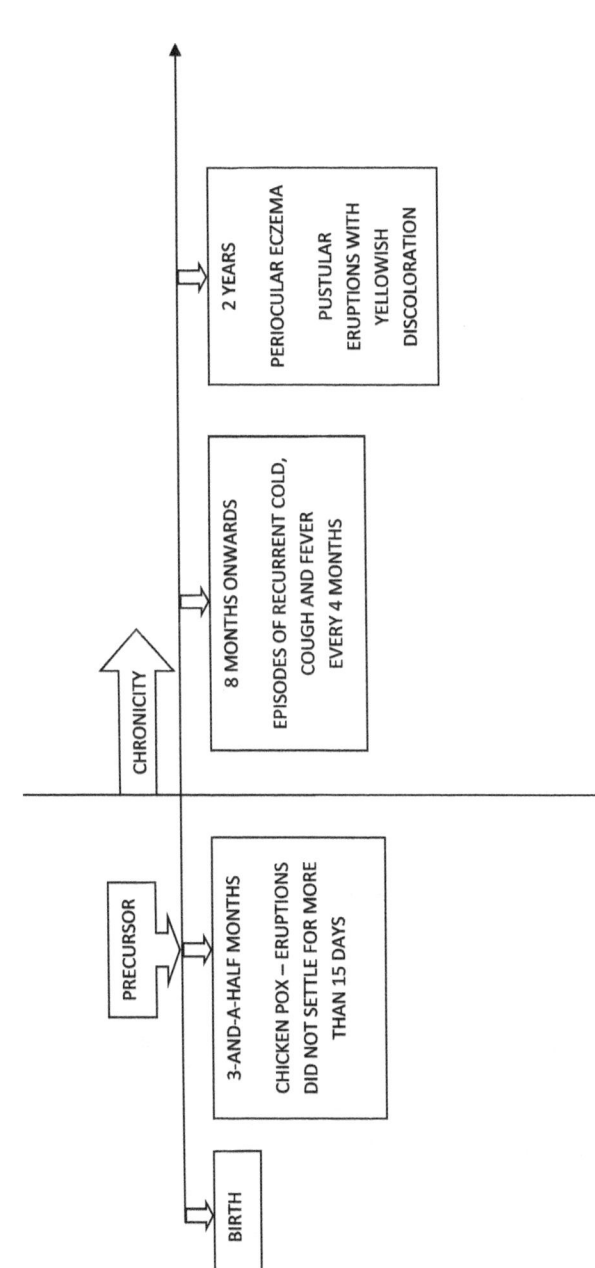

- CHRONIC MIASMATIC DISEASE – NON VENEREAL IN ORIGIN.
- Chicken Pox started the process of chronicity, further landing the patient into recurrent cold and cough and Periocular Eczema.

CHART NO. 23

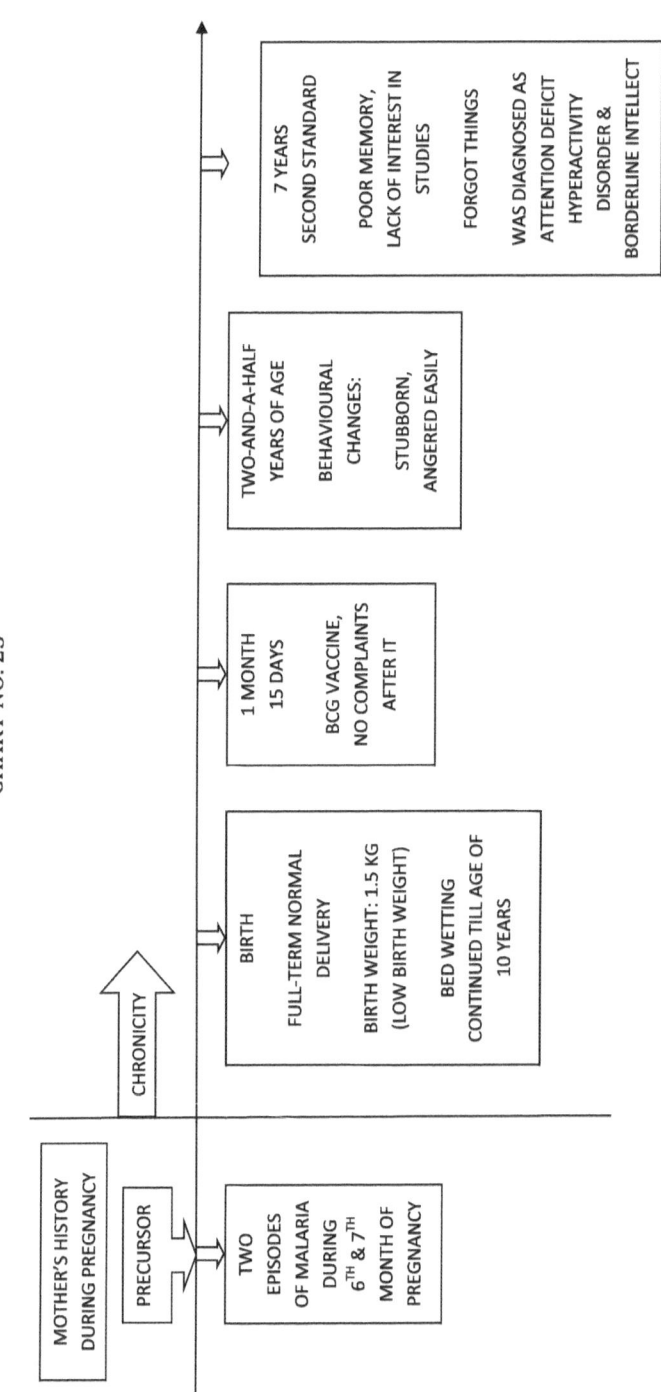

MOTHER'S HISTORY DURING PREGNANCY

PRECURSOR

TWO EPISODES OF MALARIA DURING 6TH & 7TH MONTH OF PREGNANCY

CHRONICITY

BIRTH

FULL-TERM NORMAL DELIVERY

BIRTH WEIGHT: 1.5 KG (LOW BIRTH WEIGHT)

BED WETTING CONTINUED TILL AGE OF 10 YEARS

1 MONTH 15 DAYS

BCG VACCINE, NO COMPLAINTS AFTER IT

TWO-AND-A-HALF YEARS OF AGE

BEHAVIOURAL CHANGES:

STUBBORN, ANGERED EASILY

7 YEARS
SECOND STANDARD

POOR MEMORY, LACK OF INTEREST IN STUDIES

FORGOT THINGS

WAS DIAGNOSED AS ATTENTION DEFICIT HYPERACTIVITY DISORDER & BORDERLINE INTELLECT

- **CHRONIC MIASMATIC DISEASE – NON VENEREAL IN ORIGIN.**
- The chronicity in the child appeared to be already established at birth in the form of low birth weight, the precursor being repeated malarial infection in the mother during pregnancy.
  - **EXPLANATION GIVEN IN CASE NO. 4.**

CHART NO. 24

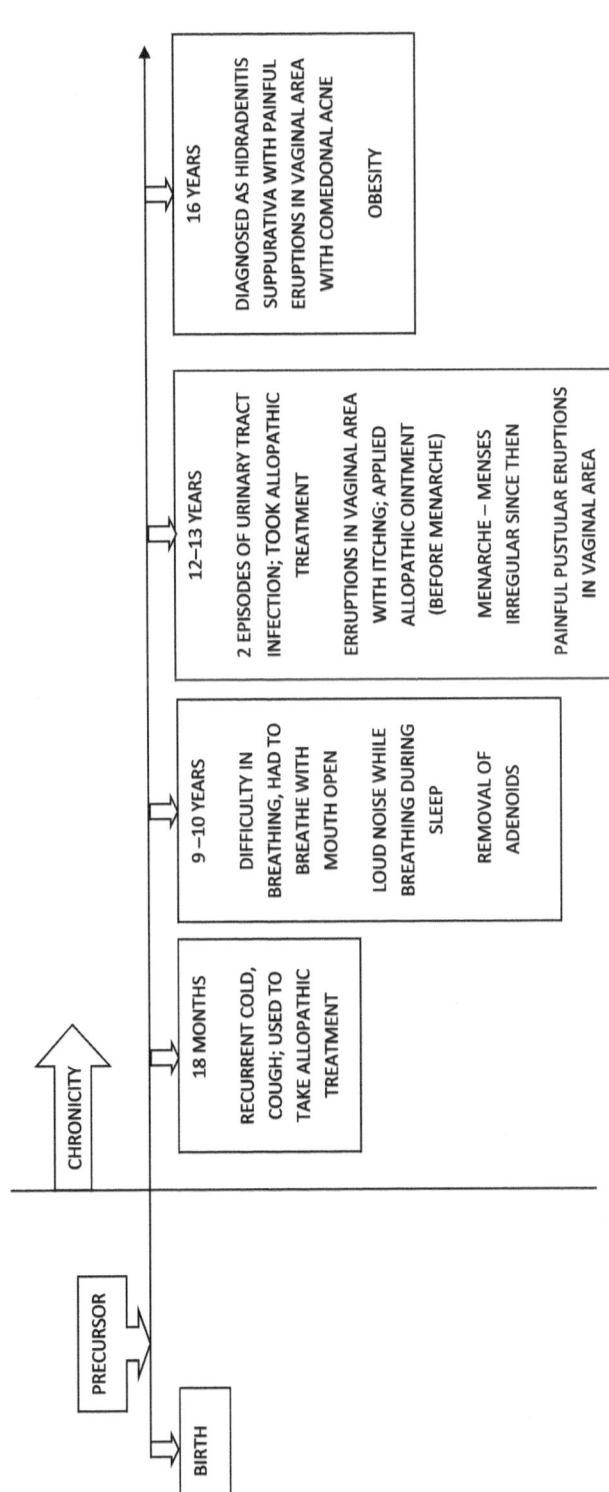

PRECURSOR

CHRONICITY

BIRTH

18 MONTHS

RECURRENT COLD, COUGH; USED TO TAKE ALLOPATHIC TREATMENT

9 –10 YEARS

DIFFICULTY IN BREATHING, HAD TO BREATHE WITH MOUTH OPEN

LOUD NOISE WHILE BREATHING DURING SLEEP

REMOVAL OF ADENOIDS

12–13 YEARS

2 EPISODES OF URINARY TRACT INFECTION; TOOK ALLOPATHIC TREATMENT

ERRUPTIONS IN VAGINAL AREA WITH ITCHNG; APPLIED ALLOPATHIC OINTMENT (BEFORE MENARCHE)

MENARCHE – MENSES IRREGULAR SINCE THEN

PAINFUL PUSTULAR ERUPTIONS IN VAGINAL AREA

16 YEARS

DIAGNOSED AS HIDRADENITIS SUPPURATIVA WITH PAINFUL ERUPTIONS IN VAGINAL AREA WITH COMEDONAL ACNE

OBESITY

- PRECURSOR NOT TRACED.
- EXPLANATION GIVEN IN CASE NO. 7.

CHART NO. 25

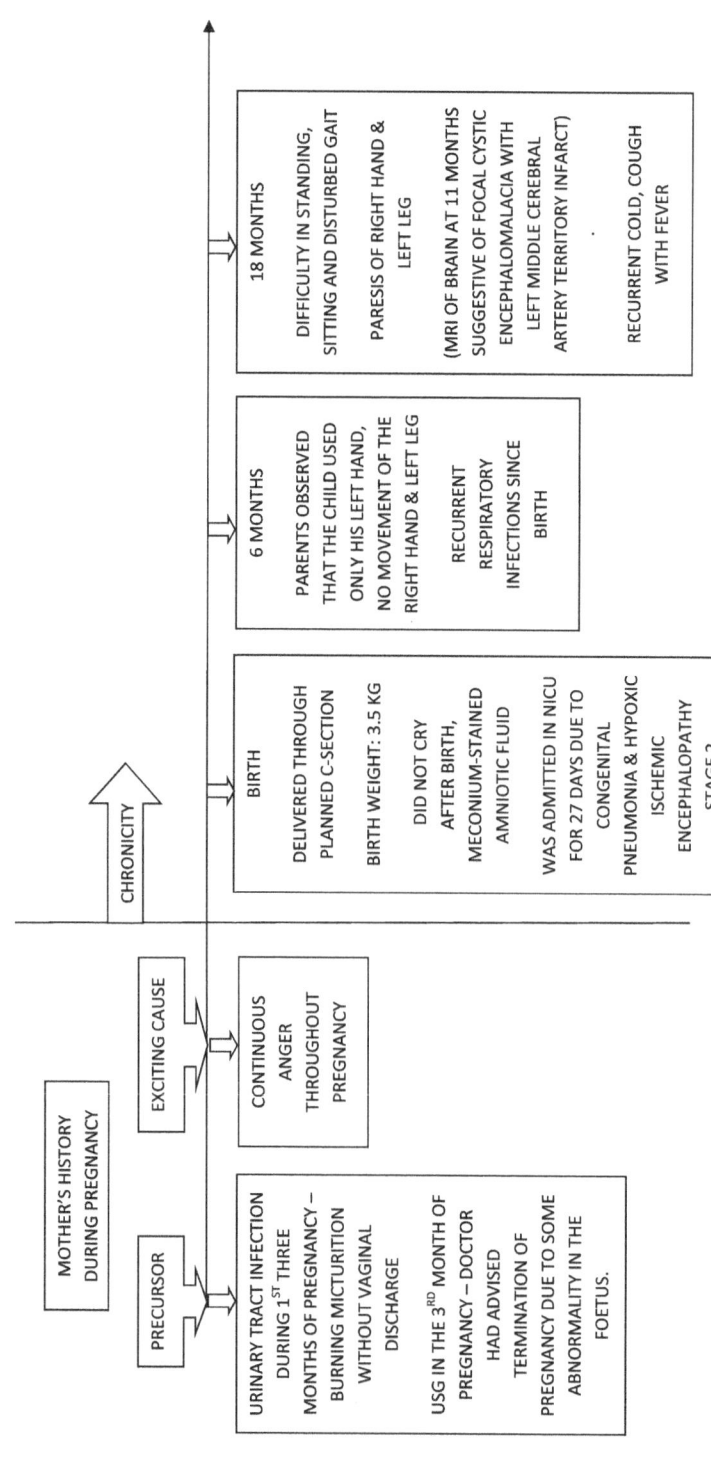

MOTHER'S HISTORY DURING PREGNANCY		

PRECURSOR

URINARY TRACT INFECTION DURING 1ST THREE MONTHS OF PREGNANCY – BURNING MICTURITION WITHOUT VAGINAL DISCHARGE

USG IN THE 3RD MONTH OF PREGNANCY – DOCTOR HAD ADVISED TERMINATION OF PREGNANCY DUE TO SOME ABNORMALITY IN THE FOETUS.

EXCITING CAUSE

CONTINUOUS ANGER THROUGHOUT PREGNANCY

CHRONICITY

BIRTH

DELIVERED THROUGH PLANNED C-SECTION

BIRTH WEIGHT: 3.5 KG

DID NOT CRY AFTER BIRTH, MECONIUM-STAINED AMNIOTIC FLUID

WAS ADMITTED IN NICU FOR 27 DAYS DUE TO CONGENITAL PNEUMONIA & HYPOXIC ISCHEMIC ENCEPHALOPATHY STAGE 2

6 MONTHS

PARENTS OBSERVED THAT THE CHILD USED ONLY HIS LEFT HAND, NO MOVEMENT OF THE RIGHT HAND & LEFT LEG

RECURRENT RESPIRATORY INFECTIONS SINCE BIRTH

18 MONTHS

DIFFICULTY IN STANDING, SITTING AND DISTURBED GAIT

PARESIS OF RIGHT HAND & LEFT LEG

(MRI OF BRAIN AT 11 MONTHS SUGGESTIVE OF FOCAL CYSTIC ENCEPHALOMALACIA WITH LEFT MIDDLE CEREBRAL ARTERY TERRITORY INFARCT)

RECURRENT COLD, COUGH WITH FEVER

- CHRONIC MIASMATIC DISEASE – NON VENEREAL IN ORIGIN.
- EXPLANATION GIVEN IN CASE NO 8.

CHART NO. 26

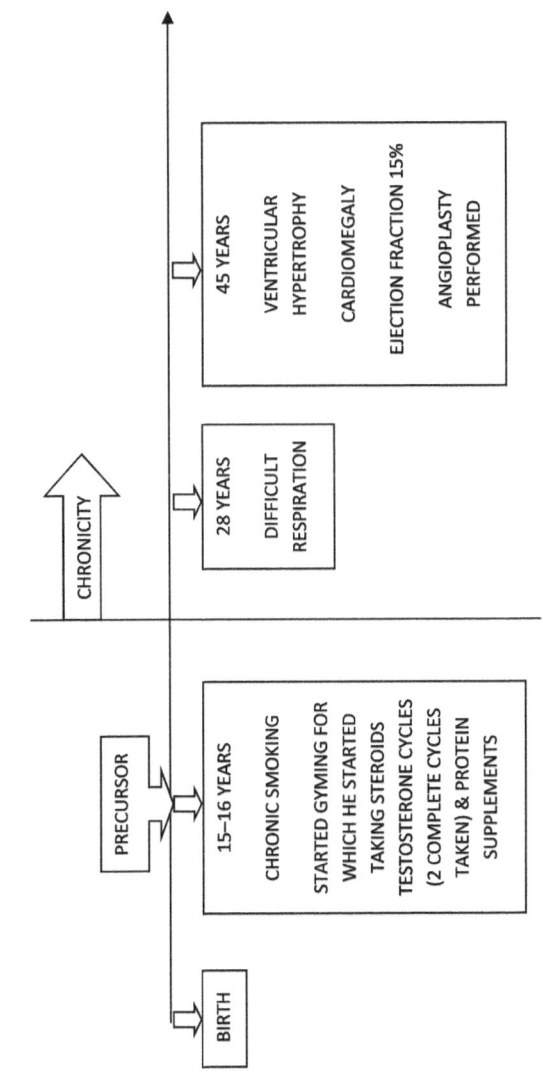

- NON-MIASMATIC ARTIFICIAL CHRONIC DISEASE.

CHART NO. 27

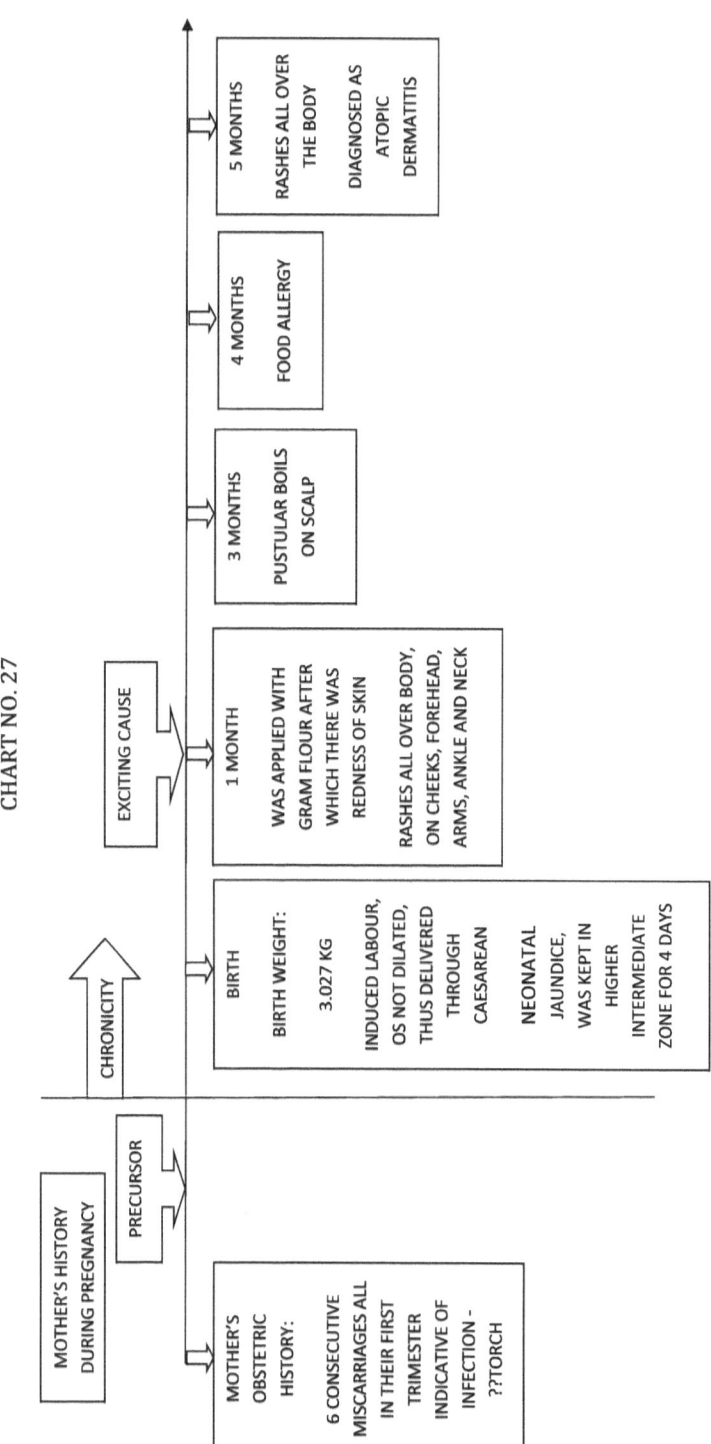

| MOTHER'S HISTORY DURING PREGNANCY | | | | | | |

PRECURSOR

CHRONICITY

EXCITING CAUSE

MOTHER'S OBSTETRIC HISTORY:

6 CONSECUTIVE MISCARRIAGES ALL IN THEIR FIRST TRIMESTER INDICATIVE OF INFECTION - ??TORCH

BIRTH

BIRTH WEIGHT:

3.027 KG

INDUCED LABOUR, OS NOT DILATED, THUS DELIVERED THROUGH CAESAREAN

NEONATAL JAUNDICE, WAS KEPT IN HIGHER INTERMEDIATE ZONE FOR 4 DAYS

1 MONTH

WAS APPLIED WITH GRAM FLOUR AFTER WHICH THERE WAS REDNESS OF SKIN

RASHES ALL OVER BODY, ON CHEEKS, FOREHEAD, ARMS, ANKLE AND NECK

3 MONTHS

PUSTULAR BOILS ON SCALP

4 MONTHS

FOOD ALLERGY

5 MONTHS

RASHES ALL OVER THE BODY

DIAGNOSED AS ATOPIC DERMATITIS

- CHRONIC MIASMATIC DISEASE – NON VENEREAL IN ORIGIN.
- The history of repeated miscarriages in the month of initial weeks of gestation indicates prevalence of infection??TORCH, which, although this baby tackled during its initial life, was soon reflected on getting triggered by application of gram flour in the form of allergy. Thus, the chronicity here was already established in the baby.
  - EXPLANATION GIVEN IN CASE NO. 6.

CHART NO. 28

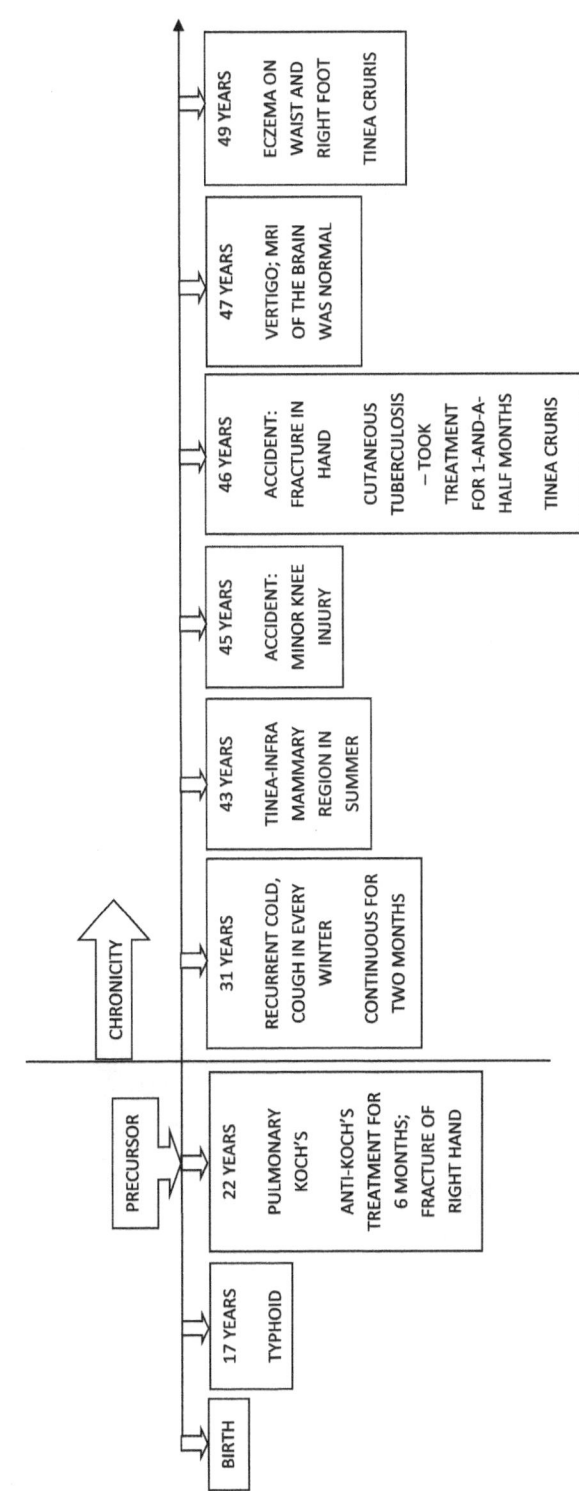

BIRTH		
17 YEARS	TYPHOID	
PRECURSOR		
22 YEARS	PULMONARY KOCH'S	ANTI-KOCH'S TREATMENT FOR 6 MONTHS; FRACTURE OF RIGHT HAND
CHRONICITY		
31 YEARS	RECURRENT COLD, COUGH IN EVERY WINTER	CONTINUOUS FOR TWO MONTHS
43 YEARS	TINEA-INFRA MAMMARY REGION IN SUMMER	
45 YEARS	ACCIDENT: MINOR KNEE INJURY	
46 YEARS	ACCIDENT: FRACTURE IN HAND	CUTANEOUS TUBERCULOSIS – TOOK TREATMENT FOR 1-AND-A-HALF MONTHS / TINEA CRURIS
47 YEARS	VERTIGO; MRI OF THE BRAIN WAS NORMAL	
49 YEARS	ECZEMA ON WAIST AND RIGHT FOOT / TINEA CRURIS	

- CHRONIC MIASMATIC DISEASE – NON VENEREAL IN ORIGIN.
- Here, Tuberculosis is the precursor, which initiated chronicity in the patient.

CHART NO. 29

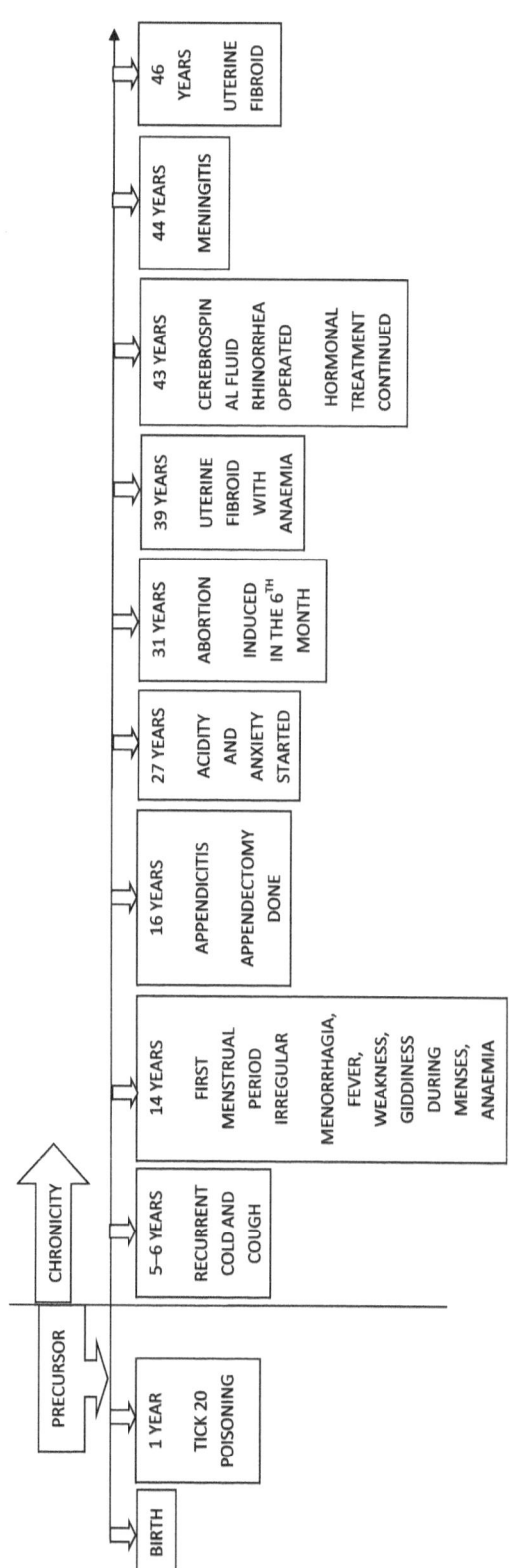

BIRTH	1 YEAR	5-6 YEARS	14 YEARS	16 YEARS	27 YEARS	31 YEARS	39 YEARS	43 YEARS	44 YEARS	46 YEARS
	TICK 20 POISONING	RECURRENT COLD AND COUGH	FIRST MENSTRUAL PERIOD IRREGULAR	APPENDICITIS APPENDECTOMY DONE	ACIDITY AND ANXIETY STARTED	ABORTION INDUCED IN THE 6TH MONTH	UTERINE FIBROID WITH ANAEMIA	CEREBROSPINAL FLUID RHINORRHEA OPERATED	MENINGITIS	UTERINE FIBROID
			MENORRHAGIA, FEVER, WEAKNESS, GIDDINESS DURING MENSES, ANAEMIA					HORMONAL TREATMENT CONTINUED		

PRECURSOR   CHRONICITY

- PRECURSOR NOT TRACED.
- Recurrent cold and cough itself signifies chronicity. Thus, a precursor before that needs to be identified, which is not traced in the above case.
- The effects of tick 20 poisoning have been eliminated from the body, as there are no residual symptoms of it.
- EXPLANATION GIVEN IN CASE NO. 5.

CHART NO. 30

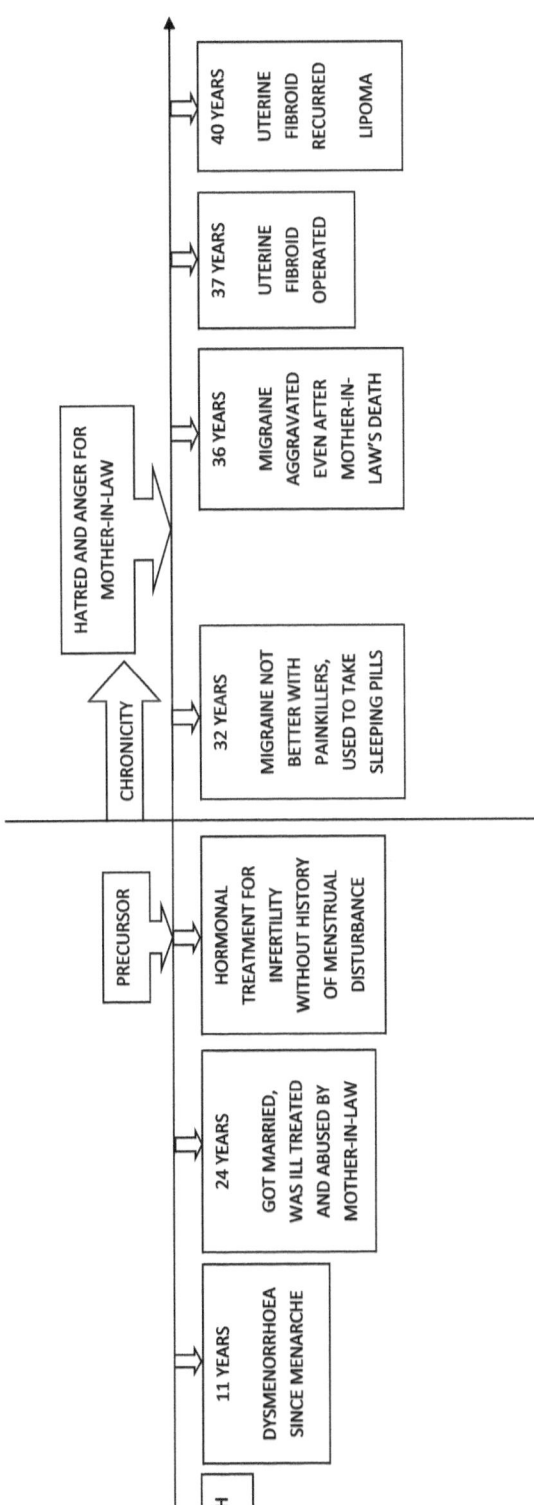

BIRTH	11 YEARS	24 YEARS	PRECURSOR	32 YEARS	CHRONICITY / HATRED AND ANGER FOR MOTHER-IN-LAW	36 YEARS	37 YEARS	40 YEARS
	DYSMENORRHOEA SINCE MENARCHE	GOT MARRIED, WAS ILL TREATED AND ABUSED BY MOTHER-IN-LAW	HORMONAL TREATMENT FOR INFERTILITY WITHOUT HISTORY OF MENSTRUAL DISTURBANCE	MIGRAINE NOT BETTER WITH PAINKILLERS, USED TO TAKE SLEEPING PILLS		MIGRAINE AGGRAVATED EVEN AFTER MOTHER-IN-LAW'S DEATH	UTERINE FIBROID OPERATED	UTERINE FIBROID RECURRED LIPOMA

- NON MIASMATIC – ARTIFICIAL CHRONIC DISEASE.
- The unnecessary hormonal treatment for a long time resulted in hormonal imbalance causing Uterine Fibroid.

STATISTICS

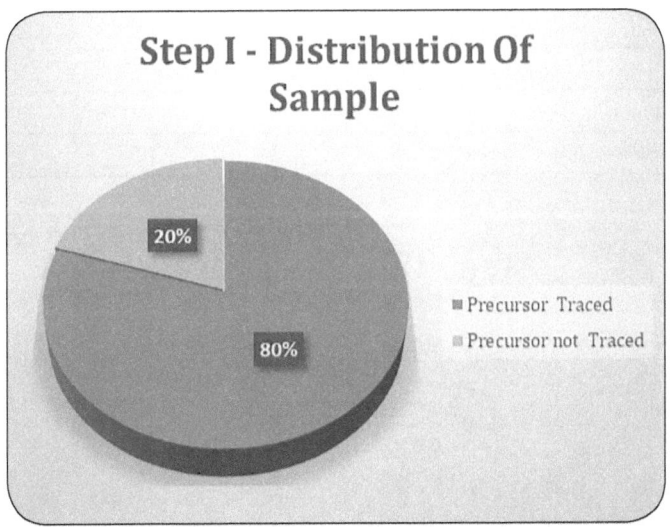

Step I - Distribution Of Sample	
Precursor Traced	24
Precursor Not Traced	6
Total	30

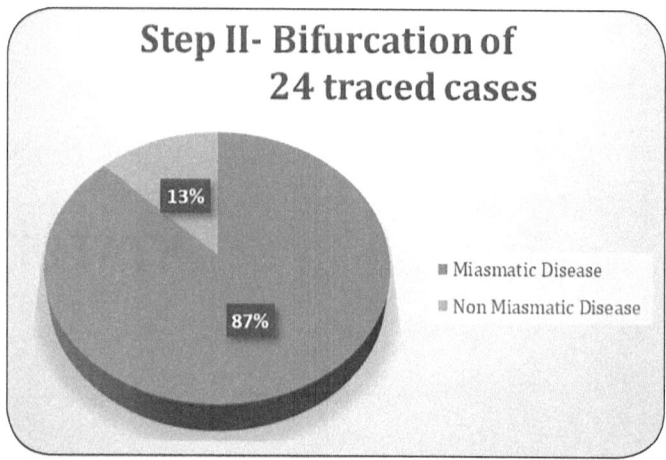

Step II - Bifurcation Of 24 Traced Cases	
Miasmatic Disease	21
Non Miasmatic Disease	3

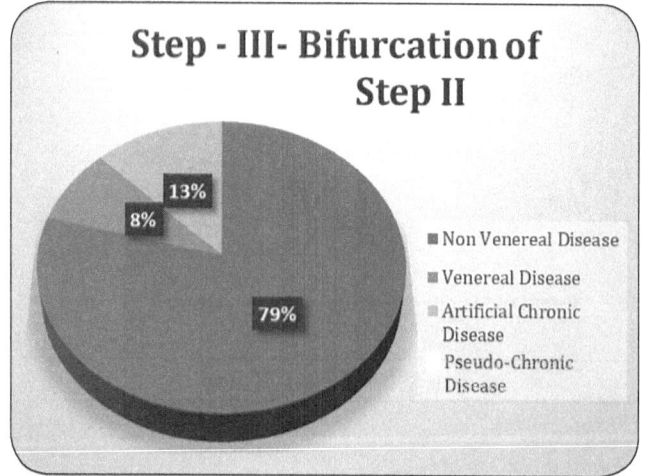

Step III - Bifurcation Of Step II	
Non Venereal Disease	19
Venereal Disease	2
Artificial Chronic Disease	3
Pseudo-Chronic Disease	0
Total	24

From the retrospective study of the journey of disease of 30 cases, we could derive the following:

> ➢ Out of 30 clinical cases, we could trace the 'precursor' in 24 cases, while in 6 cases, it remained untraced. We could attribute the failure in tracing the precursor to lack of exact details of the past ailments from the patients.
>
> ➢ Out of the 24 traced cases, the precursor was of miasmatic origin in 21 cases and of non-miasmatic origin in the remaining 3 cases.
>
> ➢ Among the miasmatic originating cases, we could attribute 2 cases to be of venereal origin and 19 cases to be of non-venereal origin.
>
> ➢ Non-miasmatic cases were further bifurcated into artificial chronic diseases and pseudo-chronic diseases.
>   - Artificial chronic diseases accounted for 3 cases.
>   - Pseudo-chronic diseases were out of sight.

Thus, we could correlate what Dr. Hahnemann had clearly mentioned in Aphorism 77 that these Pseudo-Chronic diseases are self-limiting and cannot be claimed as true chronic diseases. However, if the avoidable noxious influences persist for long, they can emerge as an artificial chronic disease. They can also uproot as a miasmatic disease, if any miasm lurks in the background.

After reviewing the writings of Dr. Hahnemann over the years, I could comprehend the distinction in case of venereal and non-venereal diseases. In non-venereal-originated diseases, the precursor enters the body and initiates the process of chronicity. Once it is initiated, the precursor is not present in the body, as it only initiates the disease process and then presents with ever-changing names and forms. Contrary to this, the precursor can always be detected in the body in case of venereal-originated diseases.

CONCLUSION

"Yet homoeopathy is a paradigmatic example of pseudoscience. It is neither simply bad science nor science fraud, but rather profoundly departs from scientific methods and theories while being described as scientific by some of its adherents (often sincerely)."

This has been affirmed by one of the renowned journals.

Since its very inception, homoeopathic science has faced numerous such censorious critics for each of its aspects. The principles of Homoeopathy, be it 'Like cures like' or even 'Law of minimal dose' have always been misapprehended, even though Homoeopathy provided a major breakthrough during the era of the so-called modern medicine. Dr. Hahnemann and the principles that he laid two centuries ago were way too ahead of their time and were misunderstood due to the fragmentary evolution of medical science.

What we today claim as prodromal symptoms have been already explained by Dr. Hahnemann that, when a patient falls sick, it is first the interior that gets affected and then the external symptoms follow. By this interior, he means not only disturbance at the level of the body but also disturbance in the smallest functional unit of the body, i.e., the cell and not ceasing here, the disturbance also disseminates to the level of proteins, which constitute a major part of our body.

Thus, Dr. Hahnemann has always guided us to, "Treat the person as a whole and not his individual parts." A man's interior gets affected by the dynamic influences which Dr. Hahnemann has already mentioned in Aphorism 11 of *Organon of Medicine* – "When a person falls ill, it is only this spiritual, self-acting (automatic) vital force, everywhere present in his organism, that is primarily deranged by the dynamic influence upon it of a morbific agent inimical to life; it is only the vital principle deranged to such an abnormal state, that can furnish the organism with its disagreeable sensations, and incline it to the irregular processes which we call disease…"

By this, we mean that the changes that occur in the temperature and pH of the environment that surrounds the proteins result from body's first defence response of inflammation. This response is the sequel of a cross reaction that occurs between the foreign protein and body's self-antigen, in case our body fails in eliminating this foreign protein from it. If these dynamic changes sustain for a prolonged time, alterations occur in the native conformation of the protein, ultimately leading to the misfolding of the proteins. As long as the protein retains its primary structure, it can refold to its normal structure and normal functioning.

All of this happens because it is only the foreign exogenous proteins that are capable of disrupting the homoeostasis of our body and predisposing it to chronicity. Thus, Dr. Hahnemann has rightly asserted that the sole culprits that produce chronic diseases are the chronic miasm, which are the foreign exogenous proteins.

These foreign proteins, as mentioned in my former book, comprise:
1. Infectious agents (Miasmatic – venereal and non-venereal)
2. Antibiotics (Non-miasmatic)
3. Chemicals (Non-miasmatic)

Although exogenous proteins have the ability to outset disease in our body, external agents such as environs, emotions, diet, etc. also play a potent role in influencing the regulatory protein and thus bring about a transformation in the expression of DNA. These factors serve as an exciter and maintainer of diseases but not the producer.

While dealing with cases in the archaic times, Dr. Hahnemann had claimed in his book *Chronic Diseases* that $7/8^{th}$ of all chronic diseases emerge from Psora (non-venereal origin) and the remaining $1/8^{th}$ arise from Syphilis and Sycosis (venereal origin).

To corroborate this even in today's era, we conducted a random study of 30 patients from a pool of around 10,000 patients visiting us, which led us to the following conclusions:

> ➤ Majority of the chronic diseases encountered were miasmatic in origin.

> ➤ Among the miasmatic originating cases, we could attribute 8% as venereal-originating and 79% as non-venereal-originating diseases.

> ➤ Among all cases, artificial chronic diseases accounted for 13%.

> ➤ Pseudo-chronic diseases were out of sight, as Dr. Hahnemann has clearly mentioned in Aphorism 77 that these Pseudo-Chronic diseases are self-limiting and cannot be claimed as true chronic diseases. However, if the avoidable noxious influences persist for long, they can emerge as an artificial chronic disease. They can also uproot as a miasmatic disease, if any miasm lurks in the background.

After reviewing the writings of Dr. Hahnemann over the years, I could comprehend the distinction in case of venereal and non-venereal diseases. In non-venereal-originated diseases, the precursor enters the body and initiates the process of chronicity. Once it is initiated, the precursor is not present in the body, as it only initiates the disease process and then presents with ever-changing names and forms. Contrary to this, the precursor can always be detected in the body in case of venereal-originated diseases.

This study thus authenticated that the teachings of Dr. Hahnemann still stay staunch in today's contemporary era. I came to fully perceive and assimilate each and every bit of this indisputable knowledge that he furnished us with, only because of the manifold experiences that my journey has unfolded. If I had not endured these experiences, it would have been difficult for me to come to terms with the theories and principles of the Founder of Homoeopathy.

Thus, quoting Albert Einstein, I also came to firmly believe that "**The only source of knowledge is experience.**"

ACKNOWLEDGEMENT

"The essence of all beautiful art is gratitude."

When I look back to this journey of my second book, it makes this belief of mine even stronger than before, when I began walking on this path. Ever since then, for me, 'I' never meant me alone. It was always 'My Team' and thus this acknowledgement is not only a gesture of my gratitude but faith towards all those because of whom this piece of literature could be accomplished. I thank The Almighty for blessing me with all the confidence, courage and sound intelligence to undertake this intended work. Also for being so merciful and kind to grant me a chance to heal his creation through this noble profession, and moreover, bestowing upon me an opportunity to spread knowledge to young minds through my experience and learning.

My immense respect and gratitude to the man of principles, humanity and knowledge, Dr. Samuel Hahnemann, the founder of Homoeopathy, for bringing into light such a wonderful science of which I am a part. The efforts of his lifetime and his quality of being far ahead of his time have been a real boon to the medical field. My intentions still remain the same as my earlier writings – to dispel the myths pertaining to Homoeopathy and establish its scientificity into today's world of advancement.

As I take this honour to present to you this literary contribution of mine, there are a few who have moulded me to what I am today, namely my teachers. I thank all my teachers who inspired and mentored me to be the best of myself right from my school years to my medical fraternity. I also take this opportunity to express my gratitude to them who expected the least from me, who may deserve this time of mine but are happily by my side living my dream all through these years. I wholeheartedly owe my gratitude to my parents, my wife and my beloved kids for sacrificing their own time and helping me accomplish my dream.

Throughout my journey from being a medical student to now being a practitioner and a teacher, one person has always been there for me whatever the circumstances were: Dr. Jayesh Dave, with whom I started just as a batch mate, then a friend, and now he is like a brother who supported me right from the foundation of our dream homoeopathic organisation to taking it ahead day by day. I am also thankful for his valuable contribution from his clinical experience through a case in this book.

I cannot forget to express my gratitude to my other friends, namely Dr. Mahesh Naik, Dr. Anil Gupta, Dr. Amruta Chaudhary, Dr. Pratiti Kothari and Dr. Divya Krishnan.

From the beginning of my journey till date, there has been a person whom I always address as my reflection and the corner stone of my credible team – Dr. Vasanth Dharmaraj. He is the first person to get an insight into any of my thoughts. Standing rock solid beside me through thick and thin, he played a significant role in bringing this forethought into reality. To team up with my work in this book, he also has a part of contribution through one of his clinical cases.

Here, I would also mention the evangelist of my team, Dr. Shridhar Boddul, who takes any task to a new horizon through his creativity and skills. Also, Dr. Lai Sangoi, who has not only contributed to this book through his clinical knowledge and discussions but has been an abiding adherent, always imparting knowledge and promoting the flourishment of this organisation.

My one family sacrificing to let me live my dream, my other family who lives this dream with me and experiences every bit of it, through all ups and downs, are my children – My Medigenites.

This book is not a work of months I would say, but for the past many years, the seed of this thought lay within me, my mind always pondering and with gradual reasoning and experiments they formed a logical interconnection.

But as they say, 'Description begins in the writer's imagination, but should finish in the reader's,' and to accomplish this, three very important people have worked day in and out to beautifully and precisely pen down my thoughts in the exact way I had compiled them in my mind. My deepest gratitude and blessings to Dr. Sneha Sharma, Dr. Namrata Ahuja and Dr. Vaidehi Mankar, for their contribution in the compilation of this book. Nobody but these people could have given the desired justice to this book.

Also, I would like to express my deep gratitude to Dr. Harshita Vora, who, since so many years, has been in close proximity with me and my work, and has been a great help to make the best of whatever I undertake. Also, special thanks to Dr. Janak Chandra for being a part of Medigene Homoeopathic International Academy and imparting knowledge to young homoeopaths.

Be it my ideas or my teachings, I always owe the credit of it to my students who have played a crucial role in this entire journey. Now when I look back at all the people who entered my life as my students and later turned out to be efficient colleagues, I feel honoured to express my gratitude to each of them personally for their valuable contribution. This list is an endless one, but each of them deserves an acknowledgement so that they know that they will always hold a special place in my heart. I owe my heartfelt gratitude to Dr. Mandeep Kaur, Dr. Sweety Soni, Dr. Hitesh Fariya, Dr. Kedar Oza, Dr. Roohee Shaikh, Dr. Purvi Mehta, Dr. Urvi Nagda, Dr. Roopal Shukla, Dr. Nikita Jain, Dr. Srushti Kotawadekar, Dr. Priyobala Thokchom, Dr. Shweta Inarkar and Dr. Neha Bharadwajan.

Last but not least, the most important people who inspire me and ignite the desire to teach within me, my Medigenites – Dr. Riddhi Shah, Dr. Hemangi Mishra, Dr. Subhashini Modali, Dr. Sagar Sonone, Dr. Nilesh Gupta, Dr. Vaishnavi Sawant, Dr. Rinki Maniar, Dr. Hitali Shah and Dr. Lohrii Charakho. I thank them for helping me grow as I learn while I teach them. My special thanks to Mr. Palashkanti Mahakur for his valuable assistance in statistical data.

To conclude, I can proudly assert: **"Team work can make a dream work!"**

BIBLIOGRAPHY

➤ *Research* at the *University of Zurich. (*31st May 2011). "Similarities cause protein misfolding"

➤ Fabrizio Chiti and Christopher M. Dobson. "Protein Misfolding, Functional Amyloid and Human Diseases". ***Annual Review of Biochemistry*** – 7 July 2006; Vol. 75:333-366

➤ Adams CL, Macleod MK, James Milner-White E, Aitken R, Garside P, Stott DI.
"<u>Complete analysis of the B-cell response to a protein antigen, from in vivo germinal centre formation to 3-D modelling of affinity maturation.</u>" *Immunology*. 2003 March; 108(3):274-87

➤ Blanden RV, Steele EJ. "<u>A unifying hypothesis for the molecular mechanism of somatic mutation and gene conversion in rearranged immunoglobulin variable genes</u>." ***Immunology and Cell Biology***. 1998 June; 76(3):288-93

➤ Boucher Y, Douady CJ, Papke RT, Walsh DA, Boudreau ME, Nesbo CL, Case RJ, Doolittle WF. "<u>Lateral gene transfer and the origins of prokaryotic groups</u>". ***Annual Review of Genetics***. 2003; 37:283-328

➤ Darwin, C.R. 1859. "On the origin of species by means of natural selection, or the preservation of favoured races in the struggle for life". London: John Murray – 1st edition

➤ Diaz M, Casali P. "Somatic Immunoglobulin Hypermutation." *Current Opinion in Immunology.* 2002 April; 14(2):235-40. Review

➤ "Heritable Integration of kDNA Minicircle Sequences from Trypanosoma Cruzi into the Avian Genome: Insights into Human Chagas Disease"

➤ *Cell,* Volume 118, Issue 2, P175-186

➤ Wu X, Feng J, Komori A, Kim EC, Zan H, Casali P. "Immunoglobulin somatic hypermutation: double-strand DNA Breaks, AID and error-prone DNA repair".

➤ *Journal of Clinical Immunology.* 2003 July; 23(4):235-46

➤ Baylin SB. "DNA METHYLATION: Tying It All Together: Epigenetics, Genetics, Cell Cycle, and Cancer." *Science.* 1997 September 26; 277(5334):1948-9

➤ *L* Pray "Epigenetics: Genome, Meet Your Environment"

➤ *The Scientist.* July 5, 2004: 14-20

➤ Watson J D, Crick F H. "Molecular structure of nucleic acids; a structure for Deoxyribose Nucleic Acid." *Nature.* 1953 April 25; 171(4356):737-8

➤ *Organon of Medicine,* Samuel Hahnemann, 6th edition, Translated by William Boericke, MD, B. Jain Publishers Pvt Ltd. 2007

➤ *The Chronic Diseases: Their Peculiar Nature and Their Homoeopathic Cure* (theoretical part) Samuel Hahnemann, translated from German, Edition by Prof. Louis. H. Tafel, Indian Books and Periodicals Publishers

➤ *Lectures on Homoeopathic Materia Medica,* Dr. James Tyler Kent, Indian Edition. Indian Books and Periodicals Publishers

➤ *The Complete Repertory,* Roger Von Zandvoort

➤ *Harrisons Principles of Internal Medicine,* Kasper, Fauci, Hauser, Longo, Jameson, Loscalzo, 20th Edition. Publisher: McGraw-Hill Education

➤ *Principles of Anatomy and Physiology,* Gerard J. Tortora, Bryan H. Derrickson, 12th Edition, John Wiley & Sons

➤ *Guyton and Hall Textbook of Medical Physiology*, John. E. Hall PhD, 13th Edition, Publisher: Saunders

➤ *Robbins Basic Pathology*, 9th edition, Vinay Kumar, Abul Abbas, Jon Aster, Harcourt Asia PTE LTD, Saunders Company

➤ *Park's Textbook of Preventive and Social Medicine*, K. Park, 23rd edition Publisher: Bhanot

➤ *Materia Medica of Homoeopathic Medicines*, Dr. S. R. Phatak, 2nd edition – revised and enlarged, 16th impression: 2013, Publisher: B. Jain Publishers (P) Ltd

NOTES

www.ingramcontent.com/pod-product-compliance
Lightning Source LLC
Chambersburg PA
CBHW021411210526
45463CB00001B/316